Manual of

3D Laparoscopy and Operative Oncology

61st AICOG BHUBANESWAR 2018

Manual of

3D Laparoscopy and Operative Oncology

Editors

SN Tripathy

KC Mahapatra

SK Giri

Prakash Trivedi

Neerja Bhatla

Sujit Behera

Manoranjan Mahapatra

JAYPEE *The Health Sciences Publisher*

New Delhi | London | Panama

Jaypee Brothers Medical Publishers (P) Ltd

Headquarters

Jaypee Brothers Medical Publishers (P) Ltd
4838/24, Ansari Road, Daryaganj
New Delhi 110 002, India
Phone: +91-11-43574357
Fax: +91-11-43574314
Email: jaypee@jaypeebrothers.com

Overseas Offices

J.P. Medical Ltd
83 Victoria Street, London
SW1H 0HW (UK)
Phone: +44-20 317 08910
Fax: +44 (0)20 3008 6180
Email: info@jpmedpub.com

Jaypee-Highlights Medical Publishers Inc
City of Knowledge, Bld. 235, 2nd floor, Clayton
Panama City, Panama
Phone: +1 507-301-0496
Fax: +1 507-301-0499
Email: cservice@jphmedical.com

Jaypee Brothers Medical Publishers (P) Ltd
17/1-B Babar Road, Block-B, Shyamoli
Mohammadpur, Dhaka-1207
Bangladesh
Mobile: +08801912003485
Email: jaypeedhaka@gmail.com

Jaypee Brothers Medical Publishers (P) Ltd
Bhotahity, Kathmandu, Nepal
Phone: +977-9741283608
Email: Kathmandu@jaypeebrothers.com

Website: www.jaypeebrothers.com
Website: www.jaypeedigital.com

Inquiries for bulk sales may be solicited at: jaypee@jaypeebrothers.com

Manual of 3D Laparoscopy and Operative Oncology

First Edition: **2018**

ISBN 978-93-5270-375-3

Printed at: Samrat Offset Pvt. Ltd.

Contributors

B Dhivya

Bhupesh Goyal
Kolkata, West Bengal

B Ramesh
Director, Altius Group of Hospitals
Bangalore, Karnataka, India

Brig Manash Biswas
Gynaecologic Oncologist,
Bangalore, Karnataka, India

Dipak Limbachiya
Ahmedabad, Gujarat

Geeta Nagasree
Hyderabad, Telangana, India

Jiten Jaipuria
Consultant, Uro-oncology division,
New Delhi, India

Rama Joshi

Rupinder Sekhon
Senior Consultant and Head,
New Delhi, India

Sabhyata Gupta
Gurgaon, Haryana, India

Shradha Chaudhari

Somashekhar SP
Bangalore, Karnataka, India

Sushil Kumar Giri
Cuttack, Odisha, India

Message

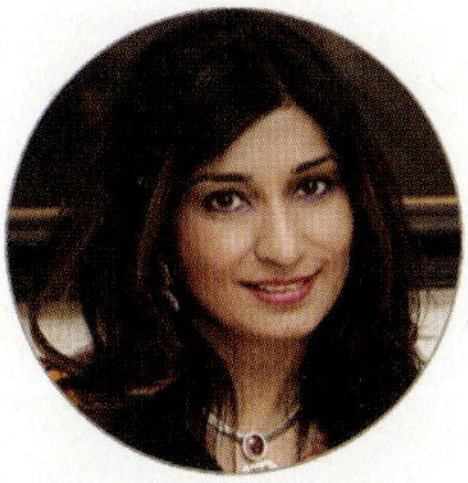

Rishma Dhillon Pai
MD DNB FCPS DGO FICOG
President, FOGSI—2017
Consultant Gynecologist
Jaslok Hospital, Lilavati Hospital and Hinduja Healthcare (Khar),
Bloom IVF Centre,
The Every Woman Clinic,
Mumbai, Maharashtra, India

"Wisdom.... comes not from age, but from education and learning."

Anton Chekhov

Life is a continuous process of learning. Especially in the field of medicine, which is constantly changing, it is very important to keep oneself abreast with the latest developments. It is heartening to note that academic workshop manuals are being released at the AICOG, Bhubaneswar, Odisha, India, for the benefit of the participating delegates and present varied updates in the field. Many different Manuals are being released on important subjects such as *3D Laparoscopy and Operative Oncology, Genetics, Fetal Medicine and Color Doppler, Postpartum Hemorrhage and High-Risk Pregnancy, Hysteroscopy,* etc.

I thank all the authors, for their immense contributions in building up the content for the manuals for Federation of Obstetric and Gynaecological Societies of India (FOGSI) by sharing their rich experiences in the field. These will be a big help to young gynecologists, who are still acquiring skills in various aspects of obstetrics and gynecology and a quick update for the seniors.

I extend congratulations to the organizing team of the AICOG 2018 and the editors of these manuals and wish you all success for this mega event.

"You cannot open a book without learning something."

—Confucius

Message

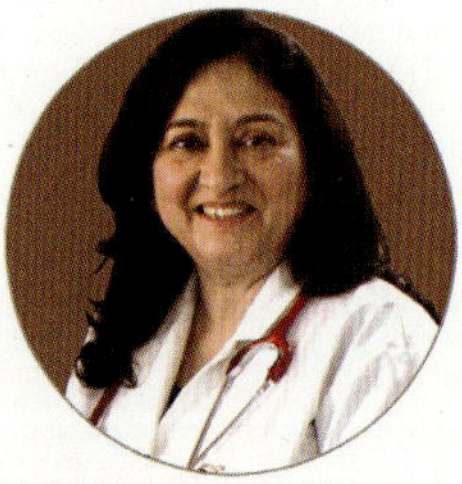

Jaideep Malhotra
MD FICMCH FICS FMAS FRCOG FICOG FRCPI FIAJAGO
Consultant ART (IVF)
President Elect, FOGSI—2018
Director, Rainbow IVF
Agra, Uttar Pradesh, India

"Education is greatest gift of life, it should never stop."

The subject of obstetrics and gynecology needs extreme proficiency as it deals with the medical specialties that focus on two different aspects. First one includes the care of pregnant women, the unborn baby, labor and delivery, as well as the immediate period following childbirth. Second aspect includes dealing with any ailment concerning the female reproductive organs. Hence, the manuals will help all those who are looking forward to gain excellence in the field of woman health. The manuals have tried to address all the issues a doctor needs.

With increasing expertise in all fields, the surgeon therefore while exercising a choice needs to follow the Hippocratic dictum—"*First, do no harm.*"

We are thankful to all those who have incorporated their contribution by providing chapters from their research and collected scientific material and have shared their fruitful experiences for the delegates of the workshop.

As a part of my agenda for 2018, I as FOGSI President 2018, plan to work actively on QED (Quality, Ethics and Dignity) among our profession and also work towards HER (Health, Empowerment and Respect) towards our patients.

"Knowledge is of no value unless you put it into practices."

Message

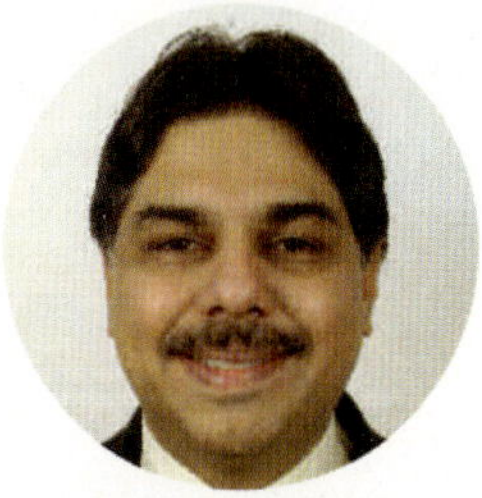

Hrishikesh Pai
Secretary General, FOGSI

It is my proud privilege to invite and welcome all delegates to the 61st All India Congress of Obstetrics and Gynaecology (AICOG) from 17th–21st January, 2018 at the Temple City of India, Bhubaneswar, Odisha, India.

It is propitious to note that the academic workshop manuals are being released which will reap beneficial reward to all the participating delegates.

I thank all the authors, for their immense contributions in building up the content for the manuals for Federation of Obstetric and Gynaecological Societies of India (FOGSI) by sharing their rich experiences in the field. These will be a big help to young gynecologists, who are still acquiring skills in various aspects of obstetrics and gynecology and a quick update for the seniors.

I forward my heartiest congratulations to all the contributors, the editors and the delegates of the workshop.

Message

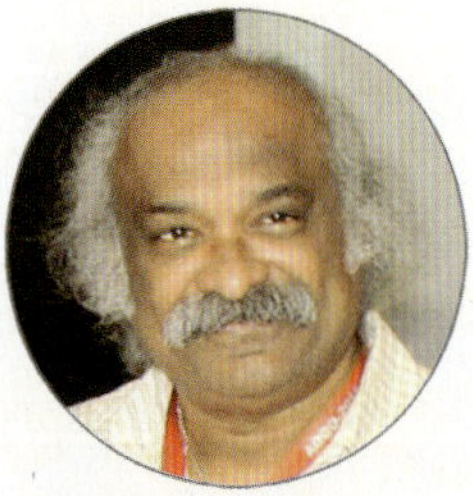

PC Mahapatra
Professor
Department of Obstetrics and Gynecology
SCB Medical College
Cuttack, Odisha, India
President, FOGSI—2011
Organising Chairperson

It is my proud privilege to invite and welcome all delegates to the 61st All India Congress of Obstetrics and Gynaecology (AICOG) from 17th–21st January, 2018 at the Temple City of India, Bhubaneswar, Odisha, India.

The five days of academic extravaganza will certainly enrich the scientific knowledge of all participating delegates and faculty. The precongress workshop on various aspects of this specialty will be held on 17th January 2018.

A quote by Edwin Louis Cole says that "*Winners are not those who never fail but those who never quit*" is apt for all the clinicians who are determined enough to see and overcome all the difficulties that are faced in the field of obstetrics and gynecology.

Today, with the advancement in the field of obstetrics and gynecology, everyone requires an in-depth knowledge of the complex subjects associated with the field so as to gain excellence in it.

This manual will prove to be a boon to all those who are associated with the field and wants to gain more knowledge in the subject matter.

Message

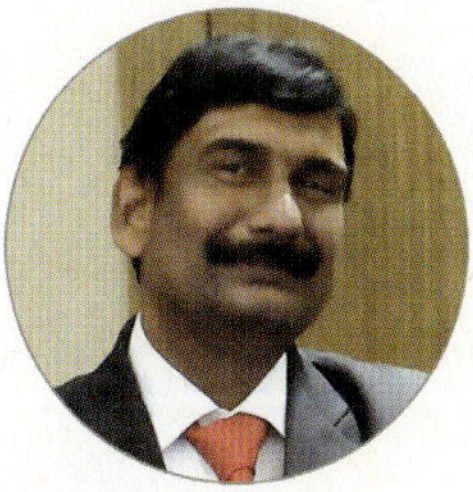

HP Pattanaik
Head
Department of Obstetrics and Gynecology
City Hospital
Cuttack, Odisha, India
Vice President, FOGSI—2009
Organising Secretary

Greetings from 61st AICOG 2018!
It is a matter of great pleasure to invite you all to 61st AICOG, from 17th–21st January, 2018 at the Temple City of India, Bhubaneswar, Odisha, India. The 11th Precongress workshops will be held on 17th January, 2018 in three medical colleges of Bhubaneswar.

It is propitious to note that the academic workshop manuals are being released which will reap beneficial reward to all the participating delegates.

It will also prove to be beneficial to the members of Federation of Obstetric and Gynaecological Societies of India (FOGSI), those who were unable to register themselves for the academic workshops.

I forward my heartiest congratulations to all the contributors, the editors and the delegates of the workshop.

Preface

'A responsible person must learn to unlearn what he has learned.'

Our branch deals with women's health from womb to tomb. So clinicians have to full knowledge and expertise to do justice to clients who trust with blind faith that they are going to get well soon at an affordable cost.

Since the introduction of the laparoscope by Jacobaeus in 1910, its usefulness in the surgical arena has been met with skepticism by traditional surgeons. Despite the skepticism, potential advantages afforded by this minimally invasive technique motivated the development and evaluation of the laparoscope in an expanding number of surgical applications. Endoscopy has now entered a golden era and almost all surgery except delivering a baby can be done by endoscopic surgery.

We have come a long way from cystoscopy to laparoscopy and 0's laparoscopy to 3D laparoscopy. A recent innovation in endoscopy is 3D laparoscopy. Dual channel endoscope creates two live-images with the camera head having two sensors. 3D vision enhances dissection and suturing by providing precise spatial orientation and reduces learning curve for young surgeons. The present standard light source is Xenon-based arc lamp, which emits light similar to daylight.

The latest addition to the armamentarium of endoscopy is the introduction of Robotic surgery. The da Vinci surgical system (US FDA Approved in 2001) is equipped with a 3-dimensional vision system. We are sure this workshop will provide and stimulate the delegates as well as the aspiring gynecologic endoscopists in aquiring knowledge regarding this important subspecialty of gynecology. Delegates will surely take home the practical tips from the stalwarts in the field of gynecological endoscopy.

Gynecological cancers remain one of the most common cancers affecting the Indian women with cervical, endometrial and ovarian cancers, constituting the majority. Surgery is the mainstay of treatment modality for gynecological cancer patients. Surgical treatment is offered with the curative intent in early stages of gynecological cancers and also advanced stages of ovarian cancers. The surgical procedures include radical hysterectomy, retroperitoneal node dissection, total omentectomy. Surgery for advanced stage ovarian cancer and endometrial cancer may include other procedures of peritoneactomy, modified posterior exenteration, bowel resection anastomosis. These surgical procedures often require a specialized skill due to complexity of the procedures to have good surgical outcome and better survival, and less morbidity and mortality. Preoperative proper assessment and good postoperative care go a long way to give maximum benefit of the surgery. To do oncosurgery one should go through a long learning curve under proper guidance. *Patient education and counseling about treatment outcomes and nutrition, lifestyle changes and about sexual health should be given to these patients.* These type of workshops also provides the same.

'I am always ready to learn although I do not always like to learn.'

—Winston Churchill

But dear friends, please learn as knowledge is power.

Editors

Content

Chapter 1

Evolution of Endovision

B Ramesh, B Dhivya

Videoendoscopy is the most common surgical procedure performed by gynecologists, colonoscopists, and gastroendoscopists, today.[1] The paradigmatic shift from open surgery into the realm of operative videolaparoscopy, took years of persistent insistence and ingenuity. It was Camran Nezhat (Fig. 1), considered the "founding father" of operative videolaparoscopy, with his visionary foresight brought this into the realm of reality.

The oldest description of endoscopic examination was in 460–375 BC where a rectal speculum was used in the Kos Scholl of Hippocrates.[2] In 500 BC, a similar speculum was described by the Babylonian Talmund.[3] Giulio Cesare Arzani in the 15th century described illumination of the rectovaginal cavities with natural light.[4]

Philipp Bozzini (Fig. 2) of Frankfurt, in 1805, used a concave mirror to reflect candle light for examining bladder and rectum.[5] Following Bozzini's idea of "magical lantern", Fisher R (United States) and Segales M (France) carried

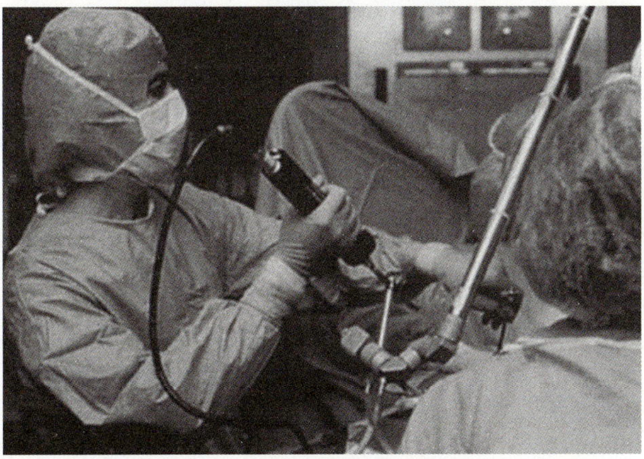

Fig. 1: Nezhat's operative videolaparoscopy (1980).

out vaginal examinations in 1805 and 1806, respectively. In 1865, Antonin Desormeaux carried out the first true endoscopy in history and presented the first "modern" cystoscope to the Academy of Medicine in Paris.[6] In 1870, Adolph Kussmaul further innovated the idea from a sword swallowing show and performed esophagoscopy with rigid tube and mirrors. In 1867, Karl Ludwig Von Bruck, a dentist created the first instrument with an internal light.

In 1877, Max Nitze, copying Von Bruck's idea, incorporated lenses, electric light and cooling system with water to the cystoscope (Fig. 3).[7]

Thomas Alva Edison's invention of the first light bulb in 1880 became a turning point in the *history of endoscopy*. However, insertion of light bulb into endoscopes resulted in numerous burns. Johann von Mikulicz-Radecki was the first to use a miniature light bulb at the end of a 30° angled gastroscope.[8] In 1887, Gustav Killian performed the first bronchoscopy with Mikulicz's instruments. In 1901, George Kelling examined the peritoneal cavity of a dog using Nitze's cystoscope and coined the term "celioscopy". In 1902, Dimitri Edler Von Ott examined the peritoneal cavity of a pregnant woman using an illuminated head mirror.[9]

The first major series of laparoscopies in humans is attributed to HC Jacobaeus. In 1910, Jacobaeus did laparoscopy using a Nitze cystoscope with "cold burning" lamps and a cannula with a valve system. He achieved his first clinical experiences in patients with ascites because puncture of the abdominal cavity appeared to be easy and without risk of inadvertent injury to intraperitoneal viscera.[10] In 1911, Bernheim, of the Johns Hopkins Medical School, reported on "organoscopy" using an ordinary proctoscope or cystoscope, with illumination from an electric headlight. He made an incision in the epigastrium, inserted the scope, and inspected the viscera and

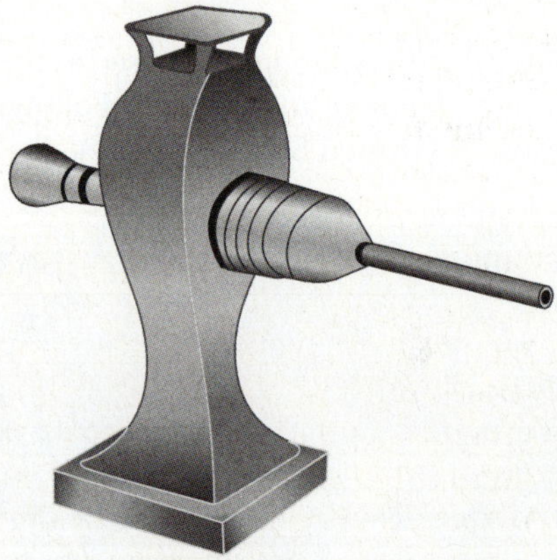

Fig. 2: Lichtleiter of Bozzini (1805).

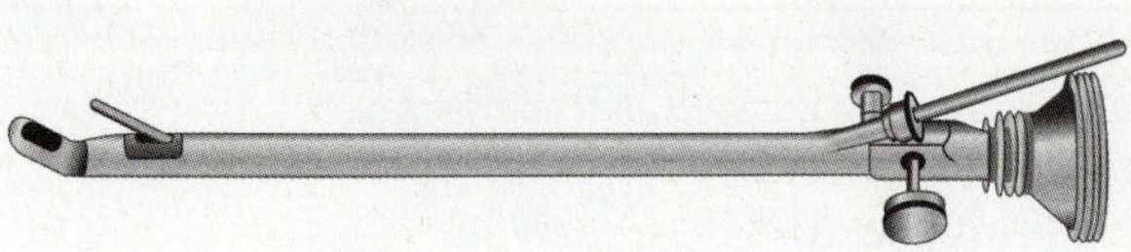

Fig. 3: Nitze's cystoscope.

drew "a part of the stomach out through the wound, made an incision in its anterior wall, and inserted the cystoscope directly into its cavity".[11] Roccavilla modified the method of illumination in 1914 and designed an instrument that permitted the source of light to remain outside the abdomen by reflecting the light through a trocar into the field of vision.[12]

In 1924, WE Stone wrote about "peritoneoscopy" in a canine model with a nasopharyngoscope through an incision in the abdominal wall and successfully completed diagnostic laparoscopies in 14 dogs with use air insufflation instead of carbon dioxide and coined the term "Laparothorakoskopie".[13] The German hepatologist Kalk, who introduced a 45° lens system, and the dual-trocar technique, which led the way to the concept of operative laparoscopy.[14] Cinematography and television had actually been used modestly in a handful of surgical centers since the late 1930s. By the 1950s, Uji, Fukami, and Suginara of Japan developed one of the earliest endoscopic cameras, the gastrocamera.[15] A new era of endoscopy began in 1952 when Fourestier et al. developed the "cold-light" fiberglass source that provided, at a low temperature, intense light through a quartz rod from the proximal to the distal end of the telescope.[16] In 1953, Cohen and Guterman introduced their Cameron cavicamera.[17] The physicist Hopkins introduced rod-shaped lenses between the glass elements to further increase illumination. This design dramatically improved the resolution and contrast of the telescope in 1953.[18] One of the most sensational moments in endoscopy's history came with the debut of Palmer's 1955 color film debut of the first live laparoscopy. In 1955, the world's first live bronchoscopy television broadcast was by Soulas and Dubois de Montreynaud.[19] Frangenheim, in 1958, produced his famous color film of a gynecologic laparoscopic surgery.[20] By 1960, Inui, Berci, and others had either invented miniaturized video endocameras into endoscopy.

Most currently used laparoscopes are designed according to the principles of the Hopkins lens system. Unfortunately until the late 1970s, these scopes were cumbersome and ineffective when the surgeon and assistant had to coordinate actions as laparoscopic visualization of the peritoneal cavity was restricted to the surgeon who held the scope. Even as late as 1977, Berci revisited the role of TV and *video devices* referred to as technologies to enhance teaching only (Fig. 4).[21,22]

Analog medical cameras have been available since the mid-1970s, but were heavy and could not be disinfected, limiting their usefulness in surgical applications. A major breakthrough occurred in 1982, when the first solid-state medical camera was introduced. Based on a silicon chip called a charge-coupled device (CCD), these digital cameras were lightweight, sterilizable, and offered improved color stability. CCDs consist of a silicon chip covered in image sensors, known as pixels, which convert incoming light energy from a visual scene into a digital signal that can be stored, processed or transmitted with greater efficiency and reliability than its analog equivalent.

Single chip cameras contain sensors for red, green and blue light embedded on a single CCD chip. Resolution of the camera is directly proportionate to the number of pixels. The resolution is defined as the amount of vertical lines that

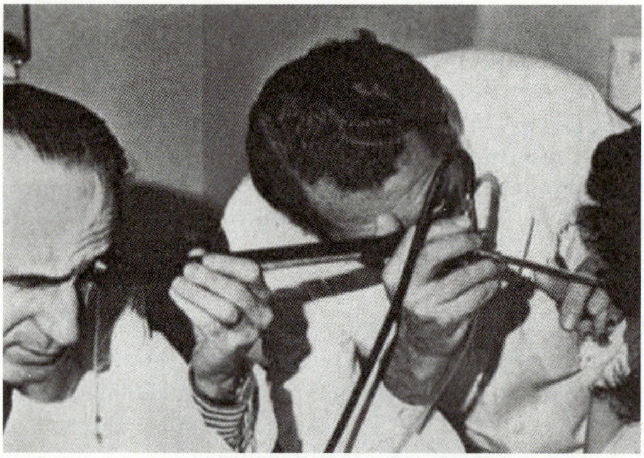

Fig. 4: Dr Berci's "teaching attachments" (1977).

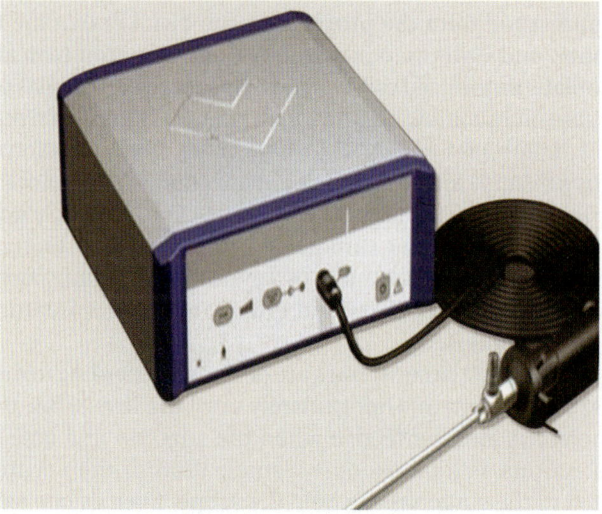

Fig. 5: Single chip camera.

may be discriminated separately in three-fourths from the width of the monitor screen. In a single chip camera (Fig. 5), multiple color sensors provided in a single chip produces videos with resolution of 400–600 lines and is adequate for routine basic surgeries. Triple chip designs utilize a prism located in the camera head unit to split the incoming image into red, green and blue components, and direct those beams of light into three separate CCD chips. The resulting image can offer superior quality in terms of color, definition and clarity, but triple chip cameras are more expensive and heavier than single chip versions. Three chip cameras (Fig. 6) have the ability of producing videos of resolution of 900–950 lines with "high quality images" and are a great help in advanced laparoscopic surgeries. A larger resolution value means a broader frequency band of the video signal. It is a measure that shows to what extent details can be distinguished on the monitor. Minimum luminance is a measure of the sensitivity of the camera to produce a good picture. Signal to noise ratio is noise to actual total video signal expressed in decibels (dB). Features of a good quality camera are higher horizontal resolution, better minimum luminance, worse signal to noise ratio.

The latest generation of cameras are high definition (HD) cameras (Fig. 7). They produce the resolution of 1,080 horizontal lines per inch, requiring HD monitors (Fig. 8) to reproduce the same quality of picture, providing a superior image with a wide, more natural 16:9 format and 1,080p resolution for full HD with two million pixels.

A recent innovation in endoscopy is three-dimensional (3D) laparoscopy (Figs. 9A to C). Dual channel endoscope creates two live images with the camera head having two sensors. Flat screen has a polarization filter and shows two images simultaneously with even-numbered-lines on screen showing image

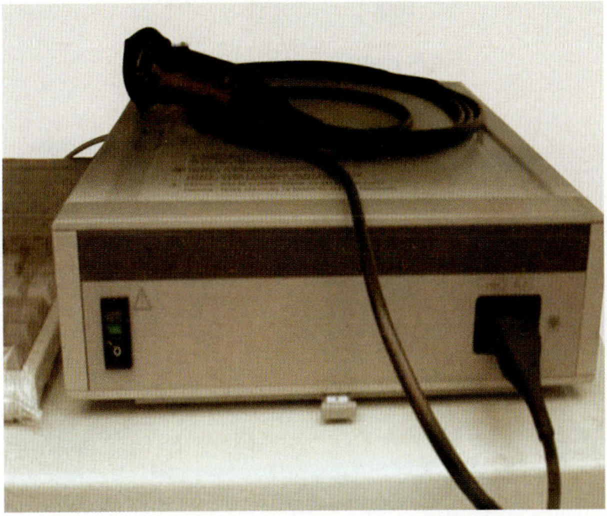

Fig. 6: Three chip camera.

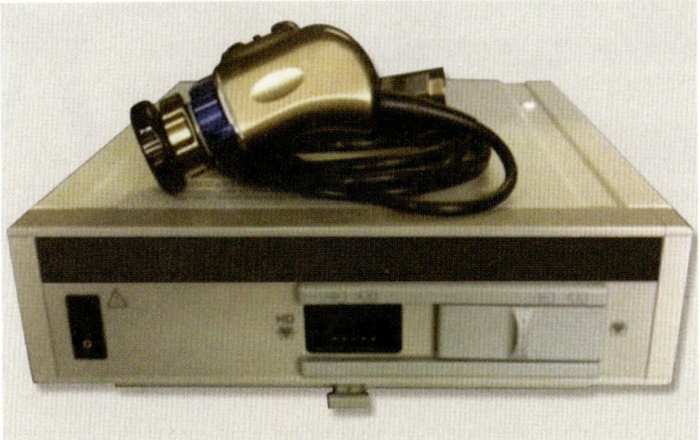

Fig. 7: High definition (HD) camera.

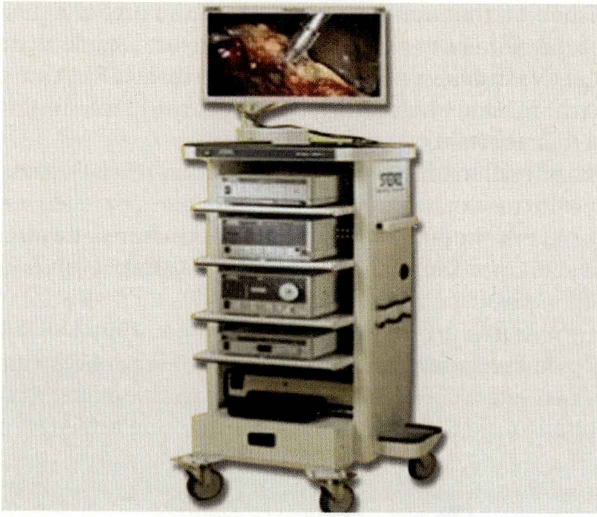

Fig 8: High definition (HD) monitor.

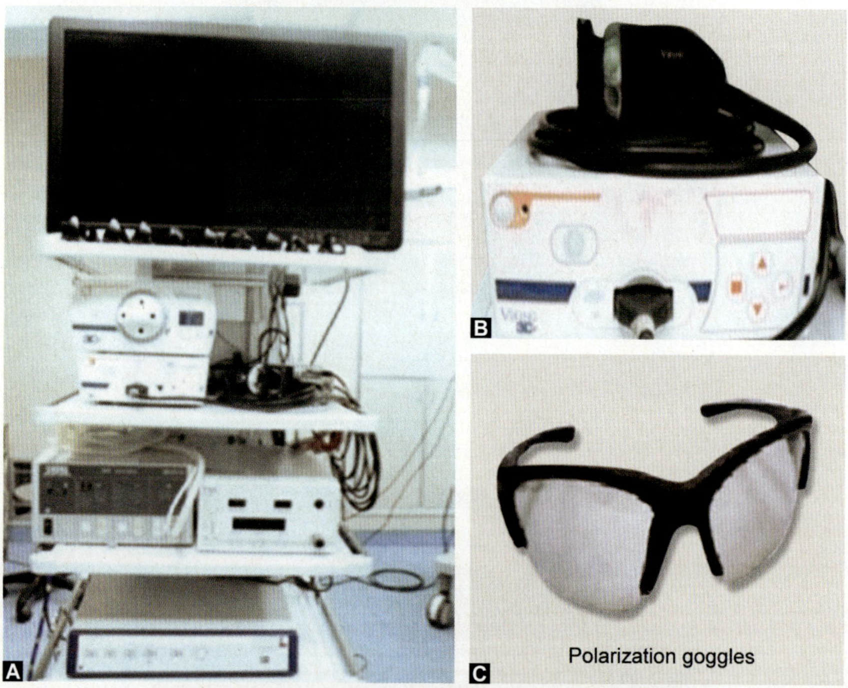

Figs. 9A to C: (A) 3D monitor. (B) 3D camera. (C) Goggles.

1, odd-numbered-lines showing image 2. Polarization glasses help sensing of image 1 by right eye and image 2 by left eye. Circular polarizing glasses separate the two images in front of the eye: the even lines can be seen only with the right eye, the odd lines can be seen only with the left eye. The human brain combines two images to one 3D impression. The displayed object seems to grow out of the flat screen resulting in true depth perception and stereoscopic visual effect. 3D vision enhances dissection and suturing by providing precise spatial orientation and reduces learning curve for young surgeons.

The latest addition to the armamentarium of endoscopy is the introduction of Robotic surgery. The da Vinci surgical system (US FDA Approved in 2001) is equipped with a 3D vision system.[23] The da Vinci robotic system has three main components: (1) the robotic cart, (2) the operating console, and (3) the endoscopic stack (Fig. 10A). The central robotic arm contains the optic system consisting of an endoscope with two optical channels and two three-chip cameras with the lateral arms holding and rotating surgical instruments freely.

The operating console integrates the 3D viewing (Fig. 10B) which improves visualization of the surgical field, thereby enhancing the precision and accuracy

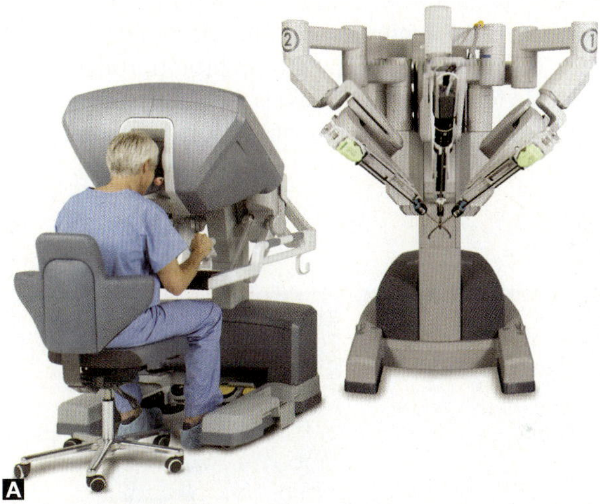

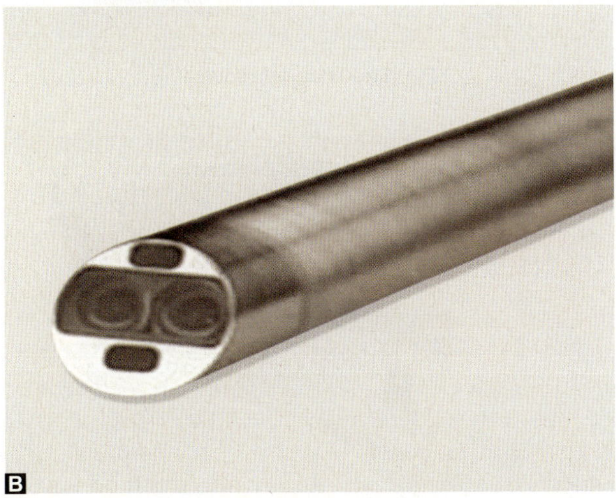

Figs. 10A and B: (A) Robotic cart with arms. (B) 3D Robotic endoscope.

of anatomic dissection. Another advantage is the wrist-like motion of the robotic arm which provides finer and more dexterous movements, enabling surgical procedures which were impossible with the conventional laparoscopy.

The present standard light source is Xenon-based arc lamp (Fig. 11), which emits light similar to day light. It deals with the use of arc based lamps, which has ergonomic challenges, lower efficiency and inability to create variety of color.

In this regard, the new generation of lighting solution is delivered by compact, inexpensive and durable high brightness light emitting diode (LED) (Fig. 12) which has better ergonomic viability. The arc-based lamps also needs to be replaced every 500 hours, while LEDs work for 50,000 hours. LEDs can produce 1,00,000 lux of illumination on operation theater table. The work by Neil Clancy et al.[24] combines the use of four spectral regions (red, green, blue and violet) using a light pipe multiplexer into a single light cable yielding a manually configurable white light at the other end. The coupling process is the key to this technology, as it may lead to high amount of loss, if coupling does not happen in a proper manner. The fluorescence imaging of protoporphyrins (which is used as a carrier molecule for divalent cations) is made possible for photodynamic diagnosis in case of bladder cancer detection by using the violet LED.

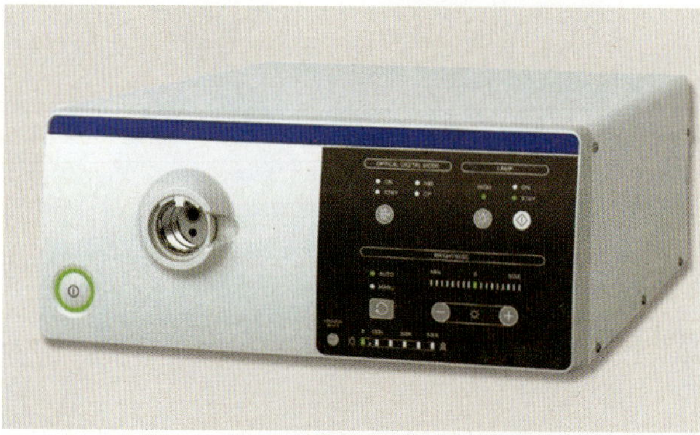

Fig. 11: Xenon light source.

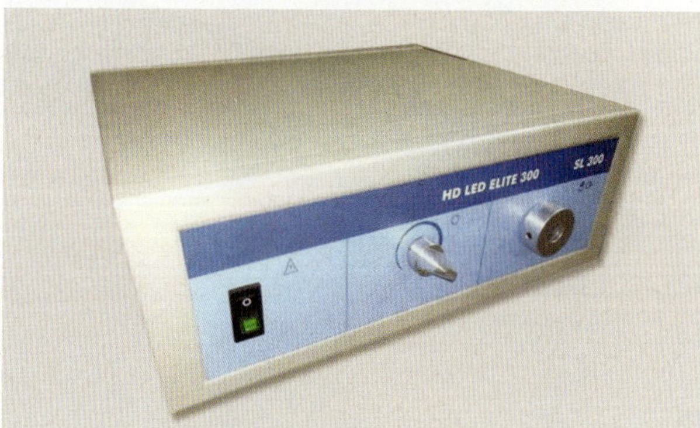

Fig. 12: Light emitting diode (LED) light source.

As stated by Lee et al.,[25] the light from LED-based systems was found to be more uniform at the distance of 4 cm with sharper shadows, higher image intensity, stable illumination despite lower radiometric power, as compared to the arc-based lamps. An example of this is narrow-band imaging (NBI), wherein, a filter wheel is moved in front of the white light source, which reduces the emitted light to two narrow bands. The blue light (415 nm) enhances the superficial capillary network, while the green light (540 nm) displays subepithelial vessels, the combination of which can be essential for certain diagnoses.

While investigating on the historical evolution of endoscopic technology, one recognizes that endoscopic equipment is used in a multitude of different application fields. Endoscopic technologies have fostered new ways of research, especially in interdisciplinary contexts. Disciplines like archeology and biology can also profit from research and developments in the medical field.

REFERENCES

1. Medina M. The trouble with trocars, quote from M. Kavic in Nov 2001. McAllen: Rio Grande Regional Hospital; 2001.
2. Lau W, Leow C, Li A. History of endoscopic and laparoscopic surgery. World J Surg. 1997;21:444.
3. Spanner SJ, Warnock GL. A brief history of endoscopy, laparoscopy, and laparoscopic surgery. J Laparoendosc Adv Surg Tech. 1997;7(6):369-73.
4. Gotz F, Pier A, Schippers E, et al. The history of laparoscopy. In: Gotz F, Pier A, Schippers E (Eds). Color atlas of laparoscopic surgery. New York: Thieme Medical Publishers; 1993. pp. 3-5.
5. Bozzini PH. Lichtleiter, ein erfindung zur anshuauung innen theile und krankheiten nebst der abbildung von Dr. Bozzini, art zu Frankfurt a. Mayn [The light conductor, an invention for viewing interior parts and diseases, with an illustration by Dr. Bozzini, physician in Frankfurt am Main]. J Pract Arzneykunde Wundarzneykunst. 1806;14:107-11.
6. Gorden A. The history and development of endoscopic surgery. Endoscopic surgery for gynaecologists. London: WB Saunders; 1993. pp. 3-7.
7. Nitze M. Eine neue Beobachtungs-und Untersuchungsmethode fur Harnrohre, Harnblause und Rectum. Wien Med Wochenschr. 1879;24:649-52.
8. Berci G, Forde KA. History of endoscopy. Surg Endosc. 2000;14(1):5-15.
9. Hatzinger M, Fesenko A, Sohn M. The first human laparoscopy and NOTES operation: Dimitrij Oscarovic Ott (1855–1929). Urol Int. 2014;92:387-91.
10. Jacobeus HC. Ueber die Möglichkeit die Zystoskopie bei Untersuchung seröser Höhlungen anzuwenden. Münch Med Wochenschr. 1910;57:2090-2.
11. Bernheim BM. Organoscopy: cystoscopy of the abdominal cavity. Ann Surg. 1911;53:764-7.
12. Roccavilla A. L'endoscopia delle grandi cavita sierose mediante un nuovo apparecchio ad illuminazione dirtta (laparo-toracoscopia diretta). La Riforma Medica. 1914;30:991-5.
13. Stone WE. Intra-abdominal examination by the aid of the peritoneoscope. J Kan Med Soc. 1924;24:63-6.
14. Kalk H. Erfahrungen mit der Laparoskopie (Zugleich mit Beschreibung eines neuen Instrumentes). Zeitschr Klin Med. 1929;111:303-48.
15. Uji T, Shirotokoro T, Hayashida T. Gastrocamera. Tokyo Med J. 1953;61:135.
16. Fourestier M, Gladu A, Vulmiere J. Perfectionnements a l'endoscopie medicale. Realisation bronchoscopique. La Presse Medicale 1952;60:1292-3.
17. Cohen M. Laparoscopy, Culdoscopy, and Gynecolography. Philadelphia: WB Saunders; 1970.
18. Gow JG, Hopkins HH, Wallace DM, et al. The modern urological endoscope. In: Hopkins HH (Ed) Handbook of Urological Endoscopy. Edinburgh: Churchill Livingstone; 1978.
19. Soulas A. Televised bronchoscopy. Presse Med. 1956;64:97.
20. Frangenheim H. Laparoscopy and Culdoscopy in Gynaecology. London: Butterworth; 1972.
21. Berci G. Present and future developments in endoscopy. Proc R Soc Lond. 1977;195:235-42.

22. Olsen V, Berci G. Teaching attachments. In: Endoscopy. New York: Appleton-Century-Crofts; 1976.
23. Kim YT, Kim SW, Jung YW. Robotic surgery in gynecologic field. Yonsei Med J. 2008;49(6):886-90.
24. Clancy NT, Sauvage V, Saso S, et al. Registration and analysis of multispectral images acquired during uterine transplantation surgery. In: Biomedical Optics and 3-D Imaging. Florida: Optical Society of America; 2012.
25. Lee AC, Elson DS, Neil MA. et al. Solid-state semi- conductors are better alternatives to arc-lamps for efficient and uniform illumination in minimal access surgery. Surg Endosc. 2009;23:518-32.

Chapter 2

Gynecological Malignancy and Laparoscopy: Yesterday's Contraindications are Today's Indications

Dipak Limbachiya

INTRODUCTION

Since the introduction of the laparoscope by Jacobaeus in 1910, its usefulness in the surgical arena has been met with skepticism by traditional surgeons. Despite the skepticism, potential advantages afforded by this minimally invasive technique motivated the development and evaluation of the laparoscope in an expanding number of surgical applications. Attempts to integrate laparoscopic techniques into the treatment of patients with gynecologic malignancies were met with an appropriate demand to show feasibility and then equivalency to traditional surgical approaches. The first case of laparoscopic staging of ovarian cancer was reported in 1975. Subsequently many others used the laparoscope as a diagnostic tool in second-look operations. The slow integration of laparoscopy into gynecology oncology, other than as a diagnostic tool, was because of the belief that radical surgery could not be performed adequately or safely. Other factors that discouraged the use of laparoscopy among gynecologic oncologists were the inability to completely evaluate the abdominal cavity due to adhesions from previous operations, the loss of tactile sense, and technical concerns such as the ability to control hemorrhage during radical surgery and lymph node dissection. Despite these concerns, many pioneering surgeons have shown the feasibility of using a minimally invasive approach in the treatment of women with gynecologic malignancies. Initially, the role of laparoscopy was limited to staging procedures. Dargent in 1987 was the first to propose the use of the laparoscope to evaluate the lymph node status, and subsequently many others reported their experiences performing laparoscopic pelvic lymph node dissections. Since then, laparoscopy applications have broadened, and instrumentation and surgical techniques have been refined.

LAPAROSCOPIC LYMPHADENECTOMY

Currently, advanced laparoscopic techniques are used to evaluate and treat cervical, endometrial and ovarian malignancies. Assessment of the invasion of the pelvic lymph nodes is a part of the staging process for these gynecological cancers. In most cases, imaging techniques cannot reliably evaluate lymphatic spread. Endoscopy offers a satisfactory means of determining the surgical stage of the disease. Pelvic lymphadenectomy can influence the therapeutic strategy, especially when a combination of treatments is proposed. Endometrial carcinoma staging requires resection of pelvic as well as para-aortic lymph nodes. The concern regarding laparoscopic lymphadenectomy is that thoroughness of dissection is not equivalent to that performed with a laparotomy. But this is of little question nowadays because of advances in technology like advent of advanced energy sources and development of 3D vision, better training and experience, which has allowed the surgeon to define retroperitoneal anatomy and complete a thorough pelvic and para-aortic lymph node dissection. Laparoscopic lymphadenectomy is one of the milestones achieved in the field of gynecological oncology as the staging and radical surgeries would stay incomplete without lymphadenectomy.

Ovarian Carcinoma

Laparoscopic surgical staging of ovarian cancer offers a number of clearly defined benefits when compared with laparotomy. Although limited, the retrospective literature examining staging for ovarian cancer confirms that the laparoscopic approach is associated with decreased estimated blood loss, shorter hospital stay, quicker return of bowel function, and shorter interval to adjuvant chemotherapy administration.

The potential pitfall is the intraoperative rupture of a malignant mass, resulting in upstaging and potentially worsening the prognosis. Therefore, it is important to make every effort to identify malignant masses before surgery, to appropriately inform and consent the patient before proceeding to exploratory laparotomy or laparoscopy. Initially laparoscopy was contraindicated because of larger sizes of ovarian masses and the risk of rupture and spillage during their retrieval. But now laparoscopy is not contraindicated, based on the risk of intraoperative rupture, as even laparotomy does not eliminate that risk nor has it been shown in a prospective fashion to even reduce it. Moreover, laparoscopy offers a unique advantage in removal of ovarian masses that are adherent posteriorly and in POD. The creation of pneumoperitoneum offers a space for dissection and adhesiolysis. Manual handling of such ovarian masses during laparotomy poses greater risk of rupture and tumor spread at the time of adhesiolysis and retrieval.

Other concern with large ovarian masses was their retrieval from abdominal cavity. But with the advent of meticulous surgical techniques and endobags, this limitation has been overcome to a large extent. The specimen after its separation from the uterus can be retrieved out by putting it in an endobag and using a minilap incision. Endobags should be used to prevent spillage of the cyst fluid content into the abdominal cavity. In cases in which the mass is too large or adherent to perform the resection without rupture, a transvaginal colpotomy may be used either to remove the intact mass or to rupture and decompress the mass while minimizing the risk of intraperitoneal spill. Using this approach, cases of successful removal of a dermoid cyst with a mean diameter of up to 10 cm have been reported.

Nowadays, laparoscopy is being used routinely for primary staging of ovarian cancers. The ability to do pelvic and para-aortic lymph node dissection as well as omentectomy to a satisfactory level using the laparoscopic approach have played a major role in shifting the mode of surgery from laparotomy to laparoscopy.

Endometrial Carcinoma

Gynecologic surgeons have been reluctant to opt for the laparoscopic approach for endometrial cancer because of following concerns. However, with the advent of new techniques and acquirement of superior surgical skills, these troubleshooters have been effectively dealt with.

First, the increased intra-abdominal pressure from CO_2 required to maintain pneumoperitoneum for a prolonged period during the operation may increase the risk of metastasis (so called port site metastasis). However, port site metastasis is estimated to occur among just over 1% of women undergoing laparoscopy for gynecological malignancy. Studies have shown this incidence to be nearly the same as that found with laparotomy scar metastasis. On the contrary, the CO_2 gas facilitates dissection by delineating tissue planes.

The other factor which might influence the slightly reduced incidence of laparotomy scar metastasis is the application of radiotherapy over the scar area as an adjuvant therapy following surgery. The incidence of port site metastasis has been shown to be reduced if the area of radiation is extended upto the port sites.

Second concern was that laparoscopic hysterectomy requires substantial manipulation of the uterus, which may increase the risk of tumor spillage and consequent dissemination. A myoma screw used to manipulate uterus to facilitate dissection may cause disruption of the cavity and disseminate tumor cells into the vagina or through fallopian tube. To overcome this, a uterine manipulator inserted per vaginam must be used.

Third issue of concern was that at the completion of laparoscopic hysterectomy, the uterus must be delivered through the vagina. Excessive manipulation, particularly of large uterus, may disrupt the wall of uterus and result in tumor spillage. But studies have demonstrated that this does not promote tumor spread. Otherwise how can hysteroscopic D&C which directly spreads the tumor cells to the intraperitoneal cavity through the distention media used via the fallopian tubes, considered the gold standard for diagnosing endometrial carcinoma. Moreover, conventional D&C which involves scrapping of endometrium also disrupts the uterine wall. However, to eliminate even this meager theoretical risk of tumor spread, the specimen must be retrieved in an endobag and then removed vaginally.

Fourth concern was the adequacy of pelvic and para-aortic lymphadenectomy. This expertise has been effectively acquired with advanced technology, experience and skills.

Cervical Carcinoma

Open radical hysterectomy had been considered the treatment of choice for early stage cervical cancer for years. In recent years, vaginal radical surgery combined with laparoscopic pelvic lymphadenectomy for early-stage cervical cancer has gained recognition in the field of oncology. Still total laparoscopic radical hysterectomy took time to gain its place because of the belief that complete parametrectomy cannot be accomplished through laparoscopy. Doubts had been raised that the thoroughness of dissection is not equivalent to that performed with laparotomy. But studies over time have proved that complete satisfactory parametrectomy can be done in an equally good way by laparoscopic approach. Despite the proven advantages of minimally invasive access for cervical cancer surgery, postoperative and long-term morbidity are considerable with regard to bladder, bowel, and sexual dysfunction due to damage of the pelvic autonomic nerves during radical hysterectomy. Nerve-sparing techniques have been introduced to preserve these structures. Identification and conservation of the inferior hypogastric plexus results in significantly less bladder dysfunction and improved sexual results, and therefore should be a mandatory approach in order to reduce surgical morbidity. Magnification during laparoscopy facilitates identification of these neural structures with measurable impact on bladder function. This offers a clear cut advantage of offering laparoscopy over laparotomy to patients with early stage cervical cancer.

CONCLUSION

Laparoscopy is selectively adopted for the management of apparently early stage disease, defined as organ-confined cancer with no evidence of gross metastatic disease, and based upon preoperative imaging studies or laparoscopic inspection.

Chapter 3

Surgical Anatomy of Uterine Cervix

Bhupesh Goyal

INTRODUCTION

Surgical anatomy of uterine cervix in a monograph on cervical cancer involves description of such anatomical facts pertaining to the cervix that will enable a pelvic surgeon to operate for cervical disease with confidence and ease. Unlike a standard textbook of anatomy, this chapter will not restrict itself to the anatomical and histological features of the cervix and its blood supply and the lymphatic drainage, but will discuss in detail the entire pelvic vascular architecture and lymphatics, nerves coursing through the pelvis likely to be encountered during extensive pelvic surgery, pelvic spaces around the cervix and the uterus, various ligaments in relation to the cervix as well as relevant description of the various vital organs in the pelvis such as urinary bladder, ureters, and rectum.

UTERINE CERVIX: ANATOMICAL FACTS

Cervix is the lower part of the uterus below the level of the isthmus. It is a fibromuscular organ, but unlike uterine corpus, it is more fibrous than muscular. Adult cervix is cylindrical in shape and measures 2.5–3.0 cm in length and about 2.5 cm in diameter. The lower half of the cervix projects into the vaginal canal and is known as the portio vaginalis. The cervix has a central canal that is bounded above by the internal os and opens into the vagina below at the external os. The cervical canal is lined by glandular epithelium whereas the portio vaginalis outside of external os is covered by stratified squamous epithelium, the more robust cover to withstand the acidic pH of the vagina. The squamocolumnar junction, which appears as the transformation zone on colposcopy, is constantly in a state of flux, moving either inward or outward, in response to the hormonal and acid-base changes in the local milieu. This metaplastic activity in the squamocolumnar junction provides the ideal soil for seeding of pathogenic viruses, such as HPV, transmitted through sexual activity, which may eventually lead to development of cancer. Squamous epithelium of the portio vaginalis is continuous with the squamous epithelium of the vaginal fornices. Bulk of the cervix comprises of cervical stroma consisting of fibromuscular, vascular and lymphatic tissues and is invested by the cervical fascia on all sides as an envelope. Muscular component of the stroma consists of loosely bound fascicles located mostly in the inner half of the cervical substance. Supravaginal portion of the cervix is in direct contact with the urinary bladder anteriorly. Posteriorly, however, it is completely covered with the visceral peritoneum, that reflects onto the rectum, forming the pouch of Douglas.

BLOOD SUPPLY

For a surgeon operating on malignant cervical disease, sound knowledge of the vascular anatomy of the pelvis, abdominal aorta downward, is an absolute must, as he would be expected to perform pelvic and para-aortic lymph node dissections in close proximity to this vascular tree.

Abdominal aorta travels along the vertebral column somewhat to the left of the midline and gives off a pair of renal arteries at the level of L1 and a pair of ovarian arteries from its anterior wall just below that. Several pairs of lumbar arteries arise from its dorsolateral aspect but are not routinely encountered during the para-aortic nodal dissection. The unpaired inferior mesenteric artery arises from its anterior aspect, 3–5 cm above the bifurcation and courses inferiorly and to the left to enter the sigmoid mesocolon. At L4 level, the aorta divides into two common iliac arteries (Fig. 1) that course inferolaterally over the sacral alae for about 4–5 cm before dividing into external and internal iliac (hypogastric) arteries. At the "V" of its bifurcation, the aorta invariably gives off the unpaired middle sacral artery that is liable to cause troublesome bleeding during the lymph node clearance if not heeded.

The *common iliac arteries* are devoid of any branches save a rather constant ureteric branch from its middle segment. *External iliac artery* (Fig. 2) courses along the lateral pelvic wall just medial to the psoas major and continues into the thigh under the inguinal ligament as femoral artery. External iliac artery does not give off any branch during its entire course except just before it goes under the inguinal ligament—the inferior epigastric artery that courses ventromedially and enters the layers of the abdominal wall. An aberrant obturator artery also occasionally arises from the external iliac artery.

Internal iliac artery (Fig. 3) lies posteromedial to the external iliac artery and courses into the depth of pelvis. This vessel supplies most of the pelvic viscera and muscles in and around pelvis. Within an inch of its origin, it gives off its posterior division that branches into a number of parietal branches to supply the pelvic and gluteal musculature. These branches are the superior gluteal, lateral sacral, and iliolumbar arteries. The anterior division of the internal iliac artery gives off at least three parietal and 5–6 visceral branches. *Uterine artery* (Fig. 4) is the first visceral branch that arises from its posteromedial aspect and

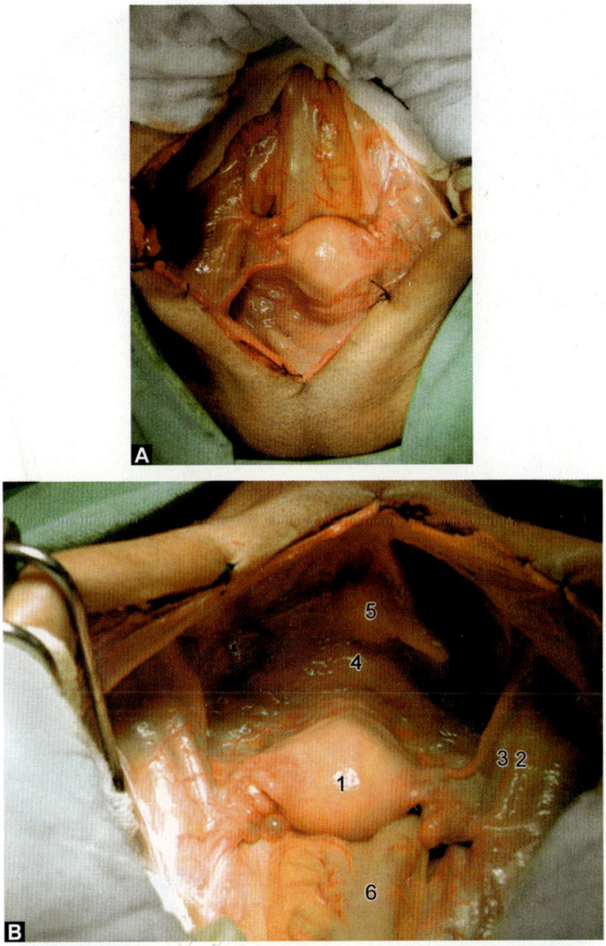

Figs. 1A and B: Pelvic anatomy after a surgical exposure (1—uterus, 2—external iliac artery, 3—external iliac vein, 4—urinary bladder, 5—Foley's catheter bulb showing through, 6—rectum).

courses anteromedially in the broad ligament to reach the isthmic region of the uterus. After the uterine artery, internal iliac artery gives off the superior and inferior vesical arteries, internal pudendal artery, inferior gluteal artery, and obturator artery before continuing anteriorly toward the umbilicus as the obliterated hypogastric artery. It is invariably possible to identify all of these branches of the internal iliac artery at extensive hysterectomy for cervical cancer.

Venous system of the pelvis comprises of a delicate network of venous tributaries spread along the pelvic walls and into the cardinal ligament that join to form the main pelvic veins. These main pelvic veins invariably accompany their corresponding arteries. There are a number of veins draining the uterus, the cervix, the vagina, and the bladder that travel behind the ureter, deep into the cardinal ligament before draining into the internal iliac vein. One or two of the smaller uterine veins, sometimes referred to as superficial uterine veins,

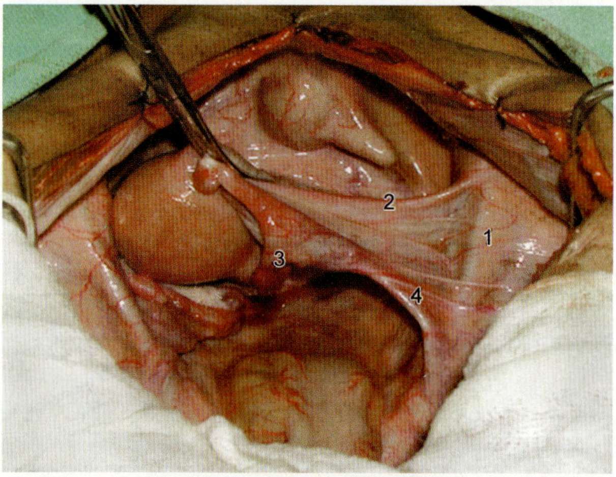

Fig. 2: Anatomical landmarks for retroperitoneal entry for pelvic nodal dissection (1—external iliac artery, 2—round ligament, 3—fallopian tube, 4—infundibulopelvic ligament).

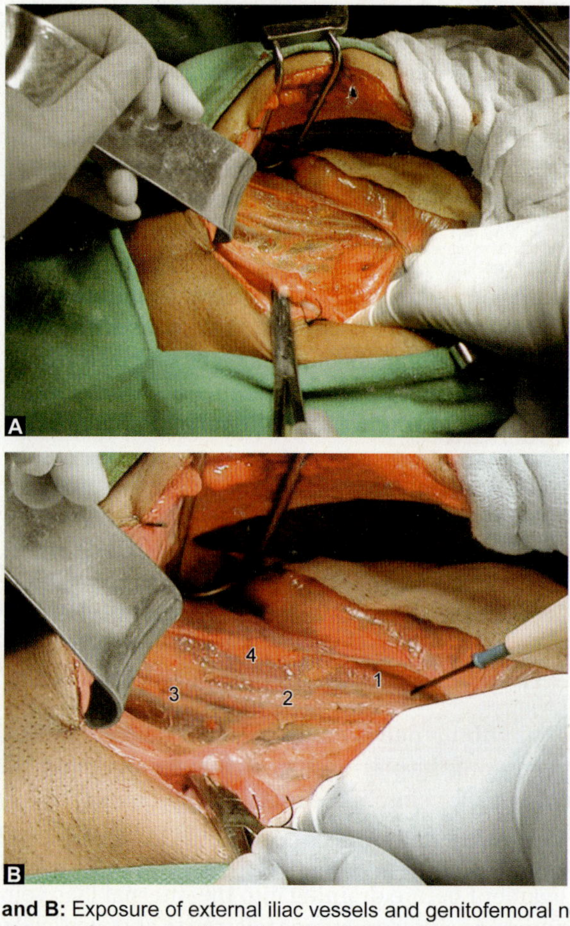

Figs. 3A and B: Exposure of external iliac vessels and genitofemoral nerve (1—genitofemoral nerve, 2—external iliac artery, 3—external iliac vein, 4—psoas muscle).

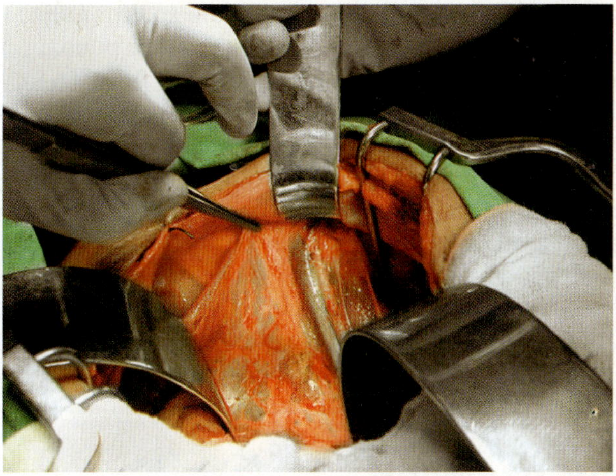

Fig. 4: Picture showing circumflex iliac vein at the caudal end of the external iliac vessels.

remain anterior to the ureter in their course to the internal iliac vein. A number of vesical veins called superior, middle, and inferior vesical veins cross in front of the ureter to empty into the deep uterine veins and require to be ligated or clipped during ureteric dissection to prevent troublesome bleeding. A network of veins draining the parieties occupies the floor and the lateral walls of the obturator fossa, deeper to the obturator nerve, that drain into the internal iliac vein. Fear of hemorrhage from these delicate venous channels in the depth of obturator fossa frequently deters gynecologic surgeons from going deeper to the obturator nerve for lymph node dissection. This may lead to incomplete nodal clearance from these sanctuary sites. It must be borne in mind that any venous bleeding deeper to the obturator nerve can easily be controlled using diathermy, ligaclips or pressure packs.

External iliac vein (Fig. 2) that starts under the inguinal ligament just medial to the external iliac artery as a continuation of the femoral vein is soon joined by a rather constant circumflex iliac vein that comes from the anterolateral direction, crossing the external iliac artery. This tributary usually marks the caudal limit of lymph node dissection along the external iliac vessels. Frequently, an accessory obturator vein drains into the caudal third of the external iliac vein posteriorly. Inadvertent injury to this vein can lead to flooding of the surgical field.

The course and relation of the right external iliac vein to external iliac artery is of particular importance to the pelvic surgeon. The vein starts medial to the artery under the inguinal ligament as stated above but courses posterior to the artery in its upper third and then crosses over to the lateral side of the external and common iliac arteries. This anatomical fact must be borne in mind when dissecting the nodes lateral to the common iliac artery.

Internal iliac vein meets the external iliac vein just caudal to the bifurcation of the common iliac artery. The axilla so formed by the fusion of these veins invariably houses nodal tissue, attempted clearance of which makes this site particularly vulnerable to trauma. The common iliac vein travels superomedially, just a little posterolateral to the corresponding artery, till its union with its fellow from the left side.

On the left side, external iliac vein stays medial to the artery throughout its course, meeting internal iliac vein to form the *common iliac vein* on left side. This vein continues inferomedial to its corresponding artery, passes under the right common iliac artery before joining the right common iliac vein to form the inferior vena cava, right lateral and a little caudal to the level of bifurcation of aorta.

A number of small tributaries drain into the inferior vena cava at various levels. Within an inch of its formation, a rather troublesome tributary joins it anteriorly. It is so vulnerable to injury by the inexperienced, that it is frequently referred to as the "fellow's vein".

LYMPHATIC DRAINAGE

Study of pattern of involvement of lymph nodes in pelvic malignancies gives a fairly good idea of the lymphatic drainage of the pelvic viscera such as uterine cervix; but at the same time also highlights the great possibility of variations from the normal in individual patients.

Lymphatics from the cervix follow the uterine vessels. Lymph channels that originate in the cervix pass through the cardinal ligament along the venous channels to go to the lymph node chains located along the external iliac artery, internal iliac artery and the obturator fossa. A few of the lymph channels pass along the uterosacrals to drain into the sacral nodes that are not easy to remove at surgery. A rather constant node is located along the uterine artery where it is crossed by the ureter.

The most caudal node along the external iliac artery, lying just beneath the inguinal ligament is the Cloquet's or Rosenmüller's node. Nodal tissue in the obturator fossa is found sheathing the obturator nerve which makes the nerve injury-prone during the obturator fossa dissection. This nodal tissue can be easily stripped from the nerve, either by retracting the external iliac vessels laterally or medially. A significant amount of fibrofatty tissue with its lymphatic channels and nodes is always seated deeper to the obturator nerve and requires to be removed in order to achieve optimum lymph node clearance in cervical cancer.

Lymphatic tissue invests the iliac vessels on all sides and is also present between the arteries and their corresponding veins. Due diligence is therefore required to remove all fibrofatty tissue from all sides of these vessels without making the vascular tree pearly white.

An important node is located in the "V" formed by the external and internal iliac veins. This node must be removed carefully at surgery to avoid trauma to the "V". Similarly, another important nodal group occupies the place just lateral to the distal common iliac artery and sitting just anterior to the common iliac vein. Attempts to remove these nodes must take care of the underlying vein.

Lymph nodes have a rich blood supply. During lymph node dissection, nodal tissue tends to ooze briskly till these are partially removed. This bleeding invariably stops without much ado once the entire lymph node bunch comes out and the feeding vessels either retract or show themselves for clipping or diathermy.

Lymphatics from the common iliac group of nodes climb along the corresponding vessels to drain into the para-aortic and paracaval group of nodes.

Nerves in the Pelvis

Pelvic surgeon operating for cervical cancer is likely to come across both somatic and autonomic nerves some of which are carefully preserved to avoid postoperative morbidity.

Genitofemoral nerve (L1, L2) (Fig. 5) is a sensory nerve that carries sensations from the anterolateral aspect of upper thigh. It courses over the psoas muscle in the pelvis, just lateral to external iliac artery, very close to the artery at times and not so close at others. Lymph node dissection at the external iliac artery always starts after identifying and saving the genitofemoral nerve, as injury to the nerve causes disturbing numbness in the upper part of thigh postoperatively.

Obturator nerve (L2, L3, L4) (Fig. 3) is a motor nerve that supplies the adductor compartment of the thigh. It enters pelvis through the belly of the psoas major just lateral to the bifurcation of the common iliac artery and courses posteromedial to the external iliac vein before exiting through the obturator canal. Along its course in the obturator fossa, it is joined by the obturator artery and vein. Damage to the nerve during clearance of the obturator fossa causes compromise of the adduction of the thigh, when specifically tested but does not cause much morbidity in the patient due to compensation by other muscle compartments.

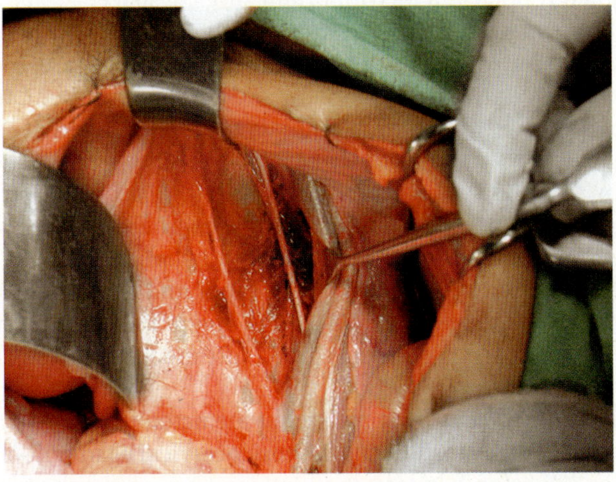

Fig. 5: Obturator fossa and obturator nerve.

Extensive dissection of the lateral common iliac nodes in the region of entry of obturator nerve into the pelvis exposes *lumbosacral plexus*, posterior to the obturator nerve. This feature is usually not sighted during surgery such extensive dissection is not routinely performed.

Sympathetic and parasympathetic nerve fibers in the pelvis accompany the vascular tree. Two discrete autonomic nerves—inferior hypogastric nerves—enter the pelvis in front of the sacral promontory and course along the posterior half of uterosacral ligaments and medial wall of pararectal space. Along its course, these nerves split into multiple fibers that go on to innervate the pelvic viscera.

PELVIC SPACES

Pelvic spaces are important anatomical features that allow the surgeon to accomplish his surgical goals with least amount of tissue trauma and intraoperative blood loss. Paravesical, pararectal, vesicouterine, and rectovaginal spaces are routinely encountered during all surgical procedures for cervical cancer. The other spaces of pelvis—retropubic space of Retzius and retrorectal space—are utilized for exenterative procedures.

Paravesical spaces (Fig. 6) are potential spaces on either side of the bladder that can be developed with ease at surgery without incurring any blood loss. Development of this space at surgery is critical as it helps in exposing the anterior aspect of the cardinal ligament and obliterated hypogastric artery. The space is bounded medially by the bladder, anterolaterally by the lateral pelvic wall (obturator internus with its overlying fascia) and pubic arch and posteriorly by the cardinal ligament. Its floor is formed by levator ani and is roofed by the parietal peritoneum. The space is usually accessed by dividing the round ligament laterally and opening the anterior leaf of broad ligament vertically downward. This exposes the obliterated hypogastric artery. Blunt finger dissection or scissor dissection lateral to the obliterated hypogastric artery completely opens up this important surgical space.

Pararectal spaces (Fig. 6) are less well-defined than the paravesical spaces and help in exposing the posterior aspect of the cardinal ligament. These spaces are bounded anteriorly by the cardinal ligament, medially by the rectum, posteriorly by sacrum and laterally by the internal iliac vessels. The floor is formed by the levator ani and is roofed by the pelvic parietal peritoneum. Care has to be exercised in developing this space to prevent unnecessary bleeding. For accessing this space, broad ligament peritoneum is opened from the divided round ligament, keeping lateral to the ureter and the infundibulopelvic ligament. With blunt and sharp dissection, loose areolar tissue of the retroperitoneal area is opened till hypogastric arteries are exposed. This space is then developed just medial to these arteries and lateral to the rectum.

Vesicocervical and vesicovaginal spaces are actually only one continuous space, separated from each other by the vesicocervical ligament—a transverse line of dense adhesion between the bladder—just above the trigone—and

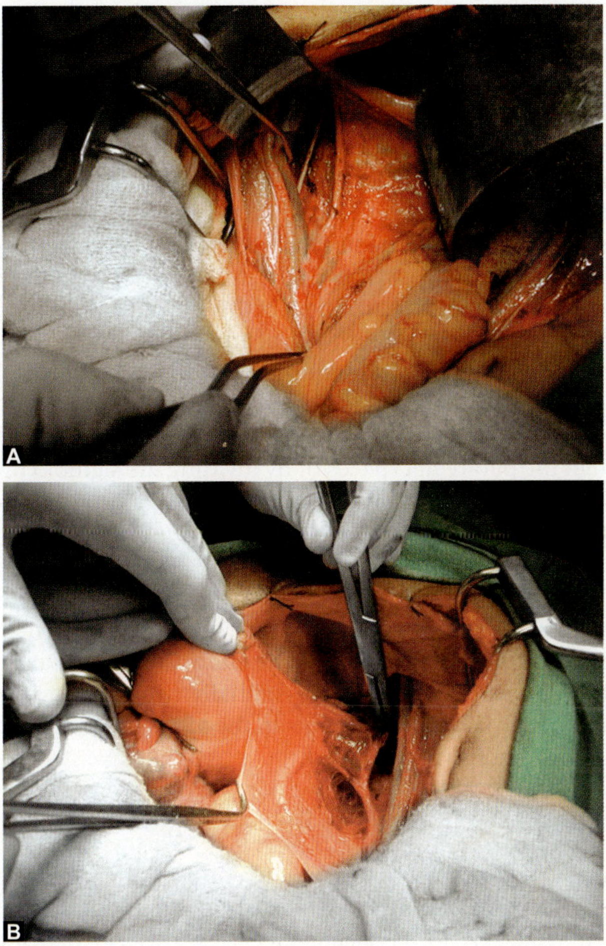

Figs. 6A and B: (A) Pelvic anatomy after completion of lymph node dissection; and (B) Uterine artery taking origin from internal iliac artery and crossing ureter.

the cervicovaginal junction. It is an avascular space with loose areolar tissue except occasional venous channels crossing the space. Vesicocervical space is bounded superiorly by the uterovesical fold of peritoneum, inferiorly by the vesicocervical ligament and laterally by the vesicouterine ligaments—the most superior portion of the bladder pillars. Vesicovaginal space is bounded laterally by the bladder pillars, inferiorly by the urogenital diaphragm and anteriorly by the bladder, urethra, and pubourethral ligaments. This vascular space allows for the separation of the bladder from the anterior vaginal wall so that adequate cuff of vagina can be developed during a radical hysterectomy for cervical cancer.

Rectovaginal space is bounded by the vagina anteriorly and rectum posteriorly. Lateral walls of this space are formed by rectal pillars which continue on to uterosacral ligament superiorly. These rectal pillars are vascular fibroconnective structures that receive the middle rectal arteries from the hypogastric artery. Inferiorly, the rectovaginal space terminates at the perineal body. This space is accessed after dividing the pouch of Douglas peritoneum and allows the development of the vaginal cuff posteriorly.

Retropubic space (Cave of Retzius) lies behind the pubic symphysis and is usually more relevant in bladder neck suspension procedures for stress urinary incontinence. In cervical cancer management, this space assumes importance during the performance of anterior exenterative procedure. This space continues with the paravesical spaces laterally, separated only by the obliterated hypogastric arteries. The floor of this space is formed by the urethra, paraurethral ligaments and urethrovesical junction.

Presacral space is bounded anteriorly by the distal portion of the sigmoid mesentery, rectum, and pararectal fossae. Posteriorly, it is bounded by the sacrum. Levator ani muscles form its inferior boundary. The space is entered either through the pararectal spaces or by dividing the sigmoid mesocolon.

LIGAMENTS

Unlike in bony joints where ligaments are well-defined, tough fibrous structures, ligaments of the pelvis are rather diffuse fibrovascular structures that are formed by the condensation of the endopelvic tissue at specific sites. The role of these pelvic ligaments is essentially two-fold: carriage of blood vessels, lymphatics and nerve elements to the visceral organs and providing them anatomical stability.

Cardinal Ligament

Also known as the lateral cervical ligament and the "web", this ligament is by far the most important anatomical structure—and frequently the waterloo—to be tackled at surgery for cervical cancer. It is described as a fan-shaped structure in the basic textbooks of anatomy, with a small medial attachment to the lateral aspect of the cervix and upper vagina and a wider posterolateral attachment to the pelvic wall and overlying vasculature. This view of the cardinal ligament obscures the fact that it is actually a 3-dimensional fan with not just an anteroposterior and side-to-side dimension but also a certain degree of height. The ligament is located at the base of the broad ligament and separates the paravesical and paravaginal spaces from the pararectal spaces. Uterine artery in its course from the hypogastric artery to the isthmus of the uterus marks the uppermost and anterior most boundary of the cardinal ligament and also represents the general direction of this ligament, almost 30° posterior to the transverse plane of the pelvis. Anterior part of this ligament contains most of the vascular elements whereas posterior part is more fibrous in form and contains the autonomic nerve supply to the bladder and rectum. Uterine vaginal inferior vesical and middle rectal arteries and veins as well as lymph nodes and lymphatics occupy this ligament.

The most important surgical fact about cardinal ligament is the traversing of the ureter through its substance that requires dissecting out and safeguarding during the course of surgery for cervical cancer. Ureter passes through the upper portion of the cardinal ligament, just beneath the uterine artery and 1–2 cm lateral to the uterine isthmus. The main uterine veins pass below the ureter but one superficial uterine vein frequently follows the artery.

Adequate central clearance at surgery for cervical cancer requires maximum removal of the cardinal ligament with all its lymphovascular contents. In surgical parlance, cardinal ligament with its contents is frequently referred to as the parametrium.

Uterosacral Ligaments

These ligaments are paired thickenings in the posterolateral pelvic peritoneum that straddle the pouch of Douglas. They originate from the posterolateral aspect of the cervix, where they are the thickest and most well-defined, and run posteriorly to the anterolateral aspect of the rectum. As they approach the rectum, these ligaments broaden such that they have a much longer attachment to the rectum than the cervix. "Uterosacral" is actually a misnomer as these are truly cervicorectal ligaments. Ureters course just lateral to the middle third of these ligaments. Since uterosacral ligaments are located in line with the rectal pillars, these are often considered the superior extensions of these structures. Autonomic nerves traverse through the posterior part of these ligaments and one method of performing nerve-sparing radical hysterectomy is to save the posterior third of the uterosacral ligaments at surgery.

Rectal Pillars

These are paired fibrovascular bundles of tissue running longitudinally between the anterolateral aspects of rectum to the posterolateral aspects of the vagina. Pararectal and paravaginal spaces are located just lateral to these structures. Rectal pillars contain extensive vascular and lymphatic connections between the vagina and the rectum. Middle rectal arteries traverse through these pillars from the cardinal ligament to the rectal wall.

Bladder Pillars

Corresponding to the rectal pillars, bladder pillars are also paired parallel longitudinal fibrovascular bundles that form the lateral limit of the vesicovaginal space and run the length of the vagina. Upper end of the bladder pillar connects to the lower half of the cervix, forming the vesicouterine ligament. The ureter passes through a tunnel in the vesicouterine ligament on its way to the inferolateral portion of the bladder wall. This divides the vesicouterine ligament into anterior and posterior leaves. Bladder pillars are often referred to as paracolpos or paravaginal tissue and contain extensive vascular and lymphatic connections between the bladder and the vagina.

Vesicouterine Ligament

Elegant description of the precise anatomy of the vesicouterine ligament was recently published by Fujii et al. Sound knowledge of the anatomy of the vesicouterine ligament makes ureteric dissection in the ureteric tunnel easier. After uterine artery is divided at its origin and lifted off the ureter medially, ureteral branch of the uterine artery and superficial uterine vein should be carefully ligated to bring into view the cranial end of the ureteric tunnel. As the connective tissue of the anterior leaf of the vesicouterine ligament is divided, a couple of small veins come into view, crossing over the ureter from lateral aspect of the cervix to the bladder. These veins are called cervicovesical veins. Once these veins are divided, the ureter is found attached to the posterior leaf of the vesicouterine ligament by certain connective tissue that is often labeled as posterior ureteral ligament. At least two small veins are found in the posterior leaf of the vesicouterine ligament. Once these veins are divided, ureters are completely mobilized from their parametrial attachments.

PELVIC VISCERA (FIGS. 7 AND 11)

Pelvic Ureter

Ureter (Figs. 1, 3, and 8 to 10) enters the pelvis at the bifurcation of the common iliac arteries just medial to the ovarian vessels in the infundibulopelvic ligament. Covered in well-vascularized adventitia, it remains retroperitoneal in position, loosely adherent to the pelvic peritoneum. Its attachment to the peritoneum is such that it is rather easy to detach it from its peritoneal attachment at surgery through a rather avascular plane. It leaves its peritoneal attachment when the parietal peritoneum on lateral pelvic wall reflects medially over the pouch of Douglas. Unlike its abdominal part, ureter in pelvis is more thick walled and can be easily identified at surgery by its cord-like feel when rolled between the thumb and the forefinger.

After it enters the pelvis, it courses somewhat posteriorly, staying anteromedial to the hypogastric artery. It then courses lateral to the middle third of the uterosacral ligament before passing under the uterine artery, 1–2 cm lateral to the uterine isthmus. It then passes through the ureteric tunnel in the vesicouterine ligament in relation to the anterolateral aspect of the vagina and finally enters the bladder base. After traversing the bladder wall for 1.5 cm, it finally opens in the bladder trigone. Its fibrovascular connections to the anterior leaf of vesicouterine ligaments are sometimes called anterior ureteral ligaments and those to the posterior leaf are called posterior ureteral ligament.

Ureter receives its blood supply from multiple sources along its journey from the renal pelvis to the bladder. In its pelvic course, it frequently gets an arterial branches from the common iliac, hypogastric, uterine and inferior and superior vesical arteries. There is an extensive anastomosing network of vessels in its adventitia that prevents segmental ischemia even if one or more of the supplying branches are severed. It is important to note that the middle third of the ureter is less well-vascularized than the upper and lower thirds.

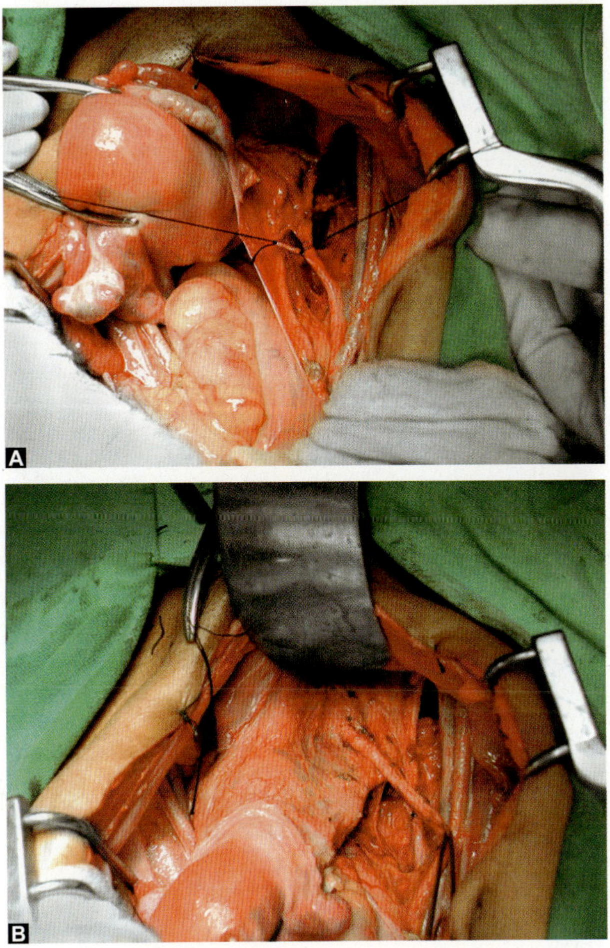

Figs. 7A and B: (A) Uterine artery ligated; and (B) Right ueretrovesical junction.

Urinary Bladder (Figs. 7 and 11)

This distensible muscular organ remains in closest contact with the female genital organs and hence vulnerable to trauma at surgery for cervical cancer. It is surrounded by potential spaces to permit distension and movement—retropubic space, paravesical spaces, and vesicocervical space. It is kept in its place by the bladder pillars and the vesicouterine ligaments, both of which are sufficiently pliant to allow great degree of distension. Dense attachment between the bladder and vagina occurs just superior to the line of trigone where it is adherent to the cervicovaginal junction (corresponding to the anterior fornix). This cervicovesical ligament separates the vesicocervical space from the vesicovaginal space. Anteriorly, the bladder neck is attached to the pubis and arcus tendineus by the pubovesical ligaments. The medial parts of these

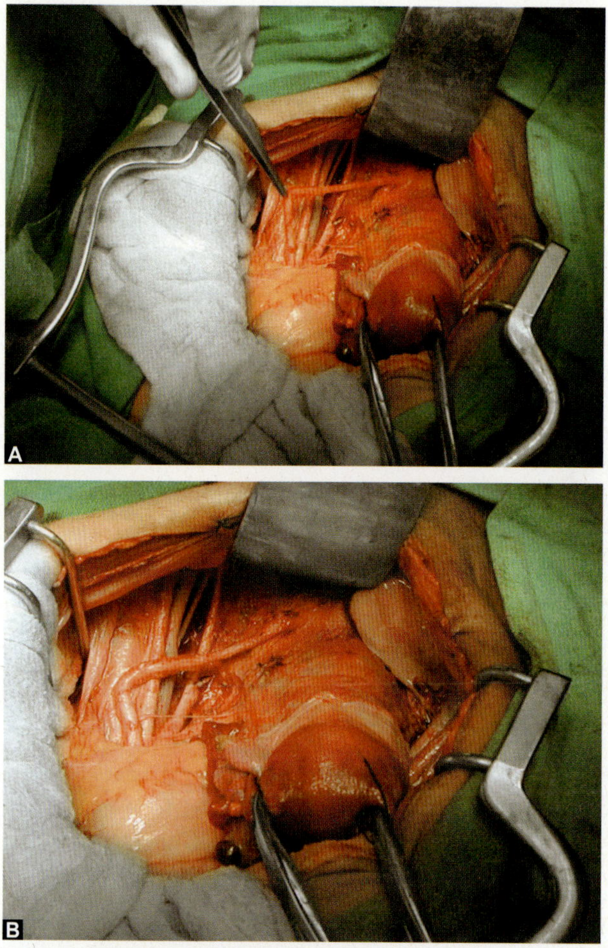

Figs. 8A and B: Left ureterovesical junction.

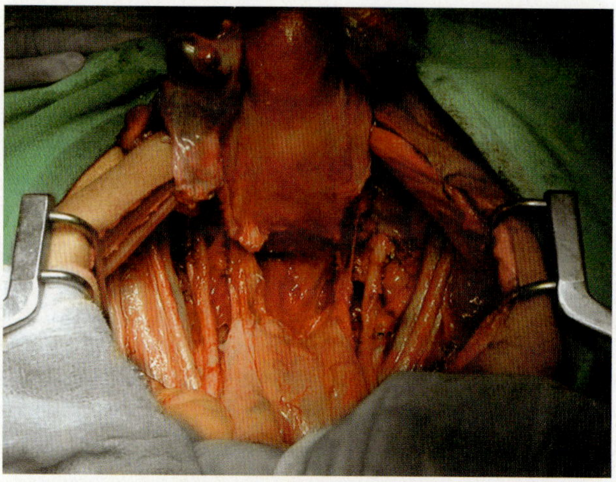

Fig. 9: Rectovaginal space.

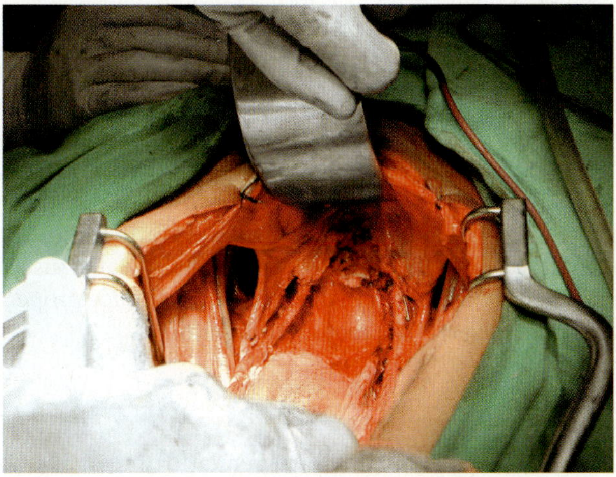

Fig. 10: Pelvic anatomy at the end of radical hysterectomy.

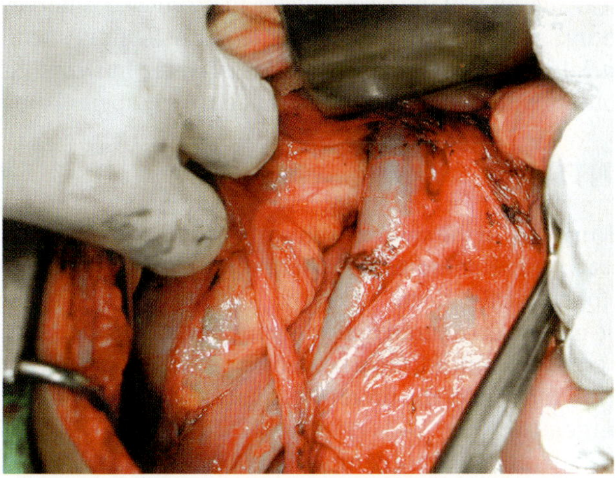

Fig. 11: Surgical anatomy of lower para-aortic area.

ligaments are much thicker than their lateral flanges. Superiorly, median umbilical ligament containing urachus extends from the dome of the bladder to the umbilicus. Additional support to the bladder comes from the pelvic floor, anterior vaginal wall and vesicourethral and pubourethral ligaments.

Bladder receives its blood supply from the obliterated hypogastric artery that gives off 1–3 superior vesical arteries and from vaginal artery that gives off inferior vesical artery. Blood supply to the bladder is abundant but richest at the bladder neck. Veins do not follow the arteries and form an extensive plexus at the base and around the bladder neck. The vesical veins have cross communication with the dorsal vein of clitoris and vaginal plexus. The vesical plexus drains into the hypogastric veins via the bladder pillars and cardinal ligaments.

Rectum (Figs. 7 and 11)

Rectum is an important posterior neighbor of the cervix, uterus and the vagina. It is covered with endopelvic fascia, known as rectal fascia that continues with the endopelvic fascia covering the levator ani. The potential space between the rectum and the vagina, the rectovaginal space is bounded on the sides by the rectal pillars and is lined by thickened endopelvic fascia. The anterior layer of this thickened fascia constitutes the rectovaginal septum (Denonvilliers' fascia) which is more adherent to the vagina than rectum. Ideally, dissection of the rectum from vagina should occur in the rectovaginal space proper, anterior to the rectal fascia to safeguard the rectum from injury.

CONCLUSION

Sound knowledge of the pelvic anatomy is essential for the surgical management of cervical cancer. Any ambiguity can result in disastrous complications for the patient, troublesome hemorrhage and great surgical strain for the operating team. Surgical anatomy of the cervix needs to be viewed differently from the pelvic anatomy as detailed in standard textbooks of anatomy, with maximum thrust on surgically relevant aspects. This chapter has highlighted these important points with their surgical relevance clearly spelled out.

KEY POINTS

- Surgical anatomy of the cervix involves not just the anatomical description of the cervix but elaborates all other pelvic features that are relevant to surgery for cervical cancer.
- It may be important to note that some insignificant anatomical facts may assume great relevance from a surgeon's point. For instance, tiny venous channels in the roof of the ureteric tunnel are of profound concern to the pelvic surgeon.
- Pelvic vasculature is highly complex and the venous system shows a high degree of variations. It is critical to be aware of this fact because veins are greatly vulnerable to trauma during surgery for cervical cancer.
- Pelvic spaces require clear understanding because radical surgery in the pelvis almost always exploits these rather avascular spaces.
- Vesicouterine ligaments and ureteric tunnel are important anatomical areas.
- Ureter, course, blood supply, relations and vulnerability must be carefully understood by pelvic surgeons because ureter must be safeguarded during radical surgery for cervical cancer.

SUGGESTED READINGS

1. Baggish MS, Karram MM. Atlas of Pelvic Anatomy and Gynecologic Surgery, 2nd edition. Philadelphia: Saunders; 2006.

2. Chi DS, Roberts CA, Abu-RustumNR. Retroperitoneal lymph node dissection. Gynecologic Oncology. 2007;104:S37-9.
3. Fujii S, Takakura K, Matsumura N, et al. Precise anatomy of vesicouterine ligament for radical hysterectomy. Gynecologic Oncology. 2007;104:186-91.
4. Morrow CP, Curtin JP, Eduardo De La Osa Lopez, et al. Gynecologic Cancer Surgery. New York: Churchill Livingstone; 1996.
5. Rock JA, Jones HW III. Te Linde's Operative Gynecology, 9th edition. Philadelphia: Lippincott Williams and Wilkins; 2003.
6. Smith JR, Priore GD, Curtin JP, et al. Atlas of Gynecologic Oncology, 2nd edition. London and New York: Taylor and Francis; 2005.

Chapter 4

Preoperative Workup of the Patients for Gyne-Oncology Surgery

Rama Joshi

INTRODUCTION

Surgery is the mainstay of treatment modality for gynecological cancer patients. Surgical treatment for gynecological cancer is offered with the curative intent in early stages of gynecological cancers and also advanced stages of ovarian cancers. The surgical procedures include the complex surgical procedures of radical hysterectomy, retroperitoneal node dissection, total omentectomy. Surgery for advanced stage ovarian cancer and endometrial cancer may include other procedures of peritoneactomy, modified posterior exenteration, bowel resection anastomosis. These surgical procedures often require a specialized skill due to complexity of the procedures also the concern of treating gynecological cancer patients often are elderly and have numerous comorbid conditions. Selection of patients and perioperative optimization of gynecological cancer patients are extremely important to ensure good surgical outcome and better survival. One of the very important factors to ensure optimal surgical outcome is to implement an operative risk assessment and to decide the best surgical treatment that poses minimum perioperative morbidity and mortality.

Surgery is performed not only with the intention to cure the diseases but in some instances also for palliative purpose. Surgery in gynecological cancer has high potential of complications. There are many vital organs and structures that are bound to be damaged or injured during the surgery such as bowel, bladder, rectum, ureters, and also pelvic vessels. Thus it is important to assess the involvement of these with proper clinical examination as well as imaging and examination under anesthetic (EUA) when indicated which will help in defining the surgical extent preoperatively. The complications can be divided into anesthetic risks and surgical risk. Aspiration, failed intubation, hypoxia, thromboembolism, respiratory and cardiovascular complications are among the important anesthetic risk. While bleeding, internal organs injuries, vascular injury, ureteric injury and sepsis are among the potential surgical risks. In addition to common surgical complications, there are few more potential complications related to specific surgical procedure such as lymphedema and lymphocele following lymphadenectomy and chronic bladder dysfunction following radical hysterectomy. Apart from physical complications, psychological, and sexual complications such as depression and sexual dysfunction could also be encountered by women following gynecological cancer surgery. Any complications that may occur will be difficult to tackle if the surgeon does not have enough experience and skill in dealing with such situation. The best clinical judgment requires experience and maturity.

Different patient may be treated by different approaches based on overall profile including the age, presence of comorbid medical problem, performance status, nature, and the extend of the disease. Surgery in gynecological cancer often requires multidisciplinary approach.

HISTORY AND PHYSICAL EXAMINATION

A thorough history and physical examination are extremely important as in most instances, majority of risk factors are discovered through good history and complete physical examination, e.g. patients on anticoagulant should stop the medication at least a week prior to surgery in order to reduce the risk of bleeding. Personal history like habit of drinking or smoking, use of contraceptives, etc. is also important. Smokers carry a higher risk of cardiovascular and pulmonary complications and surgical site infections. Family history of certain malignancies may point to a genetic basis for the disease like Lynch syndrome.

Physical examination provides information on the extent of the disease in terms of operability. Hard and fixed pelvi-abdominal mass supported with the signs of bowel or bladder invasions as well as ureteric dilatation on imaging technique always indicate difficult surgery with potentially high-risk of involvement of rectum/rectosigmoid/bladder where surgery will include modified posterior exenteration or anterior exenteration.

PATIENT WORKUP FOR DIAGNOSIS AND DISEASE STATUS EVALUATION

Contrast-enhanced computed tomography (CECT) whole abdomen and CECT chest, magnetic resonance imaging (MRI) pelvis and PET-CT whole body when indicated. Tissue diagnosis can be made through imaging guided true-cut biopsy, pleural or peritoneal fluid cytology, this is important to confirm the diagnosis and histology. Fine-needle aspiration cytology (FNAC) on ovarian mass is not recommended in the absence of extra ovarian disease and the frozen evaluation of the mass is preferred to define the malignant nature of the disease. Tumor markers based on age and provisional diagnosis like cancer antigen 125 (CA 125), cancer antigen 19-9 (CA 19-9), human epididymis secretory protein 4

(HE4), alpha-fetoprotein (AFP), lactate dehydrogenase (LDH), beta human chorionic gonadotropin (beta-HCG) and carcinoembryonic antigen, inhibin A and B, estradiol, and testosterone, are recommended. GI endoscopy and colonoscopy is sometimes considered when involvement of rectum/sigmoid is suspected. EUA, cystoscopy and rectosigmoidoscopy is done in selected advanced cervical cancer patients.

INFORMED CONSENT AND COUNSELING

Counseling regarding the present stage of disease, type of surgery and the risks involved and disease stage-based prognosis should be done properly. A thorough and well-documented consent helps to insure that the patient's expectations for her surgery, recovery, and final outcome are realistic and appropriate. The surgical team should discuss the planned procedure with the patient, and encourage her to include family or friends. Women should be approached in an open, direct, and detailed fashion; statements such as "Do not worry, I am competent enough to take care of this," or "Everything will be fine," may later lead to serious allegations if complications arise during or after surgery; no surgical outcome can be guaranteed.

PREOPERATIVE WORKUP

Basic blood investigations and urinalysis are mandatory in all patients. Chest X-ray, electrocardiography (ECG), complete blood count (CBC), liver function test (LFT), kidney function test (KFT), blood grouping, coagulation profiles is almost always required by all women undergoing major gynecological oncology surgery. Specific investigations such as echocardiogram, lung function test, etc. are indicated in selected patients. Relevant investigations of the existing comorbid condition should be considered.

OPTIMIZATION OF COMORBID ILLNESSES

Endocrine disorders like hypothyroidism, hyperthyroidism, diabetes mellitus, pheochromocytoma, and adrenal insufficiency should be normalized to the extent possible before elective surgery, whether by hormone replacement, by adrenergic blockade, or by administration of stress-dose steroids. Patient undergoing surgery following chemotherapy should be thoroughly evaluated for the effect of antineoplastic drugs on their blood count, lungs, kidneys, heart, and general condition of the patient. Cardiac patient should be referred to cardiologist for full cardiac assessment and optimization before undergoing surgery. Patient with respiratory disease should be referred to respiratory physician and they may benefit from preoperative optimizing program such us smoking caseation, use of bronchodilators, chest physiotherapy, and antibiotics.

PREOPERATIVE RISK ASSESSMENT

The most universally used classification system is the one developed by the American Society of Anesthesiologists (ASA) since 1963, which is based on the patient's functional status and comorbid conditions. The ASA index generally associates poorer overall health with increased postoperative complications, longer hospital stay, and higher mortality. Besides functional capacity and comorbid conditions, age has also been shown in some study to be a determinant of operative risk, as has the type of surgery being performed.

- Class I: Normal, healthy patient
- Class II: Patient with mild-to-moderate systemic disorder
- Class III: Patient with severe systemic disease that limits activity but is not incapacitating
- Class IV: Patient with incapacitating systemic disease that is life threatening
- Class V: Moribund patient not expected to survive 24 hours without an operation.

The most important parameter in preoperative assessment is cardiovascular and pulmonary function. While the other important parameters are age of the patient, presence of renal impairment, and endocrine dysfunction, in particularly insulin-dependent diabetes mellitus.

NUTRITIONAL STATUS

Nutritional status is a known risk factor for perioperative complication. Loss of more than 15% body weight during the previous 6 months is associated with an increased incidence of postoperative complications, including delayed wound healing, decreased immunologic competence, and inability to meet the metabolic demand for respiratory effort. Peripheral edema and signs of specific vitamin deficiencies are suggestive of severe malnutrition. Serum albumin is one of the important parameter for nutritional status and also a very important predictor for operative morbidity and mortality. Patient with severe malnutrition should be referred to a dietician and should receive nutritional therapy before and after surgery. Patient with poor bowel functions and those who are unable to consume food orally for more than 5 days should be subjected for parenteral nutrition.

The patients undergoing the gyne-oncology surgery require detailed assessment for disease extent, proper metastatic workup and preoperative workup to optimize the surgical outcome.

Chapter 5

Venous Thromboembolism in Gynecological Cancers

Geeta Nagasree

INTRODUCTION

Deep vein thrombosis (DVT) and pulmonary thromboembolism (PTE) together constituting *venous thromboembolism (VTE)* is a major complication of gynecological malignancies causing major morbidity and mortality. VTE can either present as an initial clinical presentation, or as a complication of surgery for gynecological malignancies. The exact incidence of VTE ranges between 3% and 25%. The difference is seen due to the differences in the methods of diagnosis used in the various studies. The incidence is more in studies using the Iodine^{125} fibrinogen leg scans, while the incidence is less in studies taking purely clinical criteria. In the postoperative patient, VTE was significantly more likely after gastrointestinal, lung, prostate, and ovarian/uterine operations with an associated mortality over six times. Iodice et al. reported a meta-analysis in which the pooled relative risks (RR) of VTE versus no VTE were significantly elevated for the cancers of the ovary (RR 7.0), pancreas (RR 6.1), liver (RR 5.6), blood (RR 4.2), brain (RR 3.8), kidney (RR 3.4), lung (RR 3.1) and colon (RR 2.9).

The risk of thrombosis in cancer is increased four times, and for those undertaking chemotherapy, the incidence rises up to 6.5 times. Venous thromboembolic disease is the second leading cause of death among cancer patients and raises cancer related morality 2–8 times. The rate of VTE in cancer patients is slowly increasing over the past 6 years, possibly reflecting the widespread use of new procoagulant drugs. The stage of the disease also seems to have an impact on the incidence of the disease, with greater incidence in more advanced stages. For patients presenting with more than one risk factor besides cancer, the overall VTE rate is high: 40–80% will present distal DVT, 10–20% will present proximal DVT, 4–10% will have clinical PTE, and 1–5% will present fatal PTE.

PATHOPHYSIOLOGY OF VENOUS THROMBOEMBOLISM

The Virchow's triad described by Virchow in 1858 forms the basis of the pathophysiology of patients presenting with venous thromboembolism (VTE). Trousseau reported that cancer was associated with thrombophlebitis. The risk of VTE can be further due to either the disease characteristics, patient related characteristics or the therapeutic or iatrogenic characteristics. The Virchow's triad proposes the causal relation of venous thrombosis included endothelial injury, stasis of blood flow and activation of the clotting factors. Several tumor factors or patient factors can cause disruption of the triad. In addition, the change in the components of the triad can be seen as a manifestation of the pathophysiological processes of the malignancy itself. Endothelial injury can be caused by the various tumor-induced factors such as tissue factors, reduced thrombomodulin, thrombospondin, tissue pathway inhibitor and altered angioprotein 2/-1 proportion. Venous stasis can be caused by the tumor mass itself, extrinsic compression or the increased secretion of procoagulants. Activation of procoagulant pathways can be caused due to secretion of procoagulants and reduction of natural coagulation inhibitors. The formation of the blood clots further promotes the growth of the cancer cells and facilitates the spread of cancer. Perioperative factors too may play an important part such as immobility, pelvic masses causing compression and stasis of blood, injury to various vessels due to surgical dissection or indwelling lines and catheters, ingrowths of tumors, use of procoagulant drugs, increased hematocrit and dehydration, and formation of a procoagulant state.

DIAGNOSIS

- The clinical presentation of VTE comprising of DVT and PTE ranges from mild dyspnea to sudden cardiac death.
- Dyspnea is the most common symptom. An index of suspicion is needed as dyspnea in a postoperative patient can be due to several reasons such as basal atelectasis, anemia, pain, indwelling drains or tubes. Patient may also present with increased anxiety or restlessness.
- There can be occasional chest pain or cough.
- Tachycardia and tachypnea should be distinguished from other causes such as pain, anxiety, anemia, dehydration and fever.
- Lungs on evaluation may be normal; the second heart sound may sometimes be accentuated. There can be syncope or sudden cardiac death.
- Signs and symptoms of DVT include lower extremity swelling, and that lower limbs may be warm to touch and tender.
- Timely treatment and high clinical suspicion is essential as the mortality may be 5–7%.
- Wells' clinical decision rule for DVT helps in the diagnosis of DVT. The criteria are scored as follows:
  - Clinical symptoms of DVT (3 points). Other diagnoses less likely than PTE (3 points)

- Heart rate greater than 100 beats/min (1.5 points)
- Immobilization for at least 3 days or surgery in previous 4 weeks (1.5 points)
- Previous DVT/PTE (1.5 points)
- Hemoptysis (1 point)
- Malignancy (1 point).

- In the modified Wells criteria, PTE is likely when the score is greater than 4 and unlikely when the score is less than 4. Highly sensitive D-dimer is coupled into the decision algorithm.
- Common conditions to differentiate from DVT include cellulitis, lymphedema, vein compression, hematoma, and trauma. PTE should be differentiated from CHF, basal atelectasis, anemia and myocardial infarction.

LABORATORY INVESTIGATIONS

- Room air ABG shows hypoxemia, respiratory alkalosis, and alveolar oxygen disproportionately higher than arterial oxygen levels.
- D-dimer indicates activation of fibrinolysis. It is highly sensitive and has a high negative predictive value. Values of D-dimer less than 500 ng/mL rules out PTE.
- Other markers associated with and having prognostic value include Troponins, Brain Natriuretic Peptide (BNP) and N terminal Pro-BNP.
- Chest radiographs are often normal. Some of the abnormal findings may be reduced pulmonary vascularity (Westermark's sign), elevation of diaphragm (Hampton hump) and infiltrates or pleural effusion.
- Computerized tomography angiography scan has a high sensitivity and specificity where the embolus is seen as a filling defect. It has 95% predictive value. The scan is technically inaccurate or inadequate in about 1–10% of cases.
- Doppler ultrasonography show thrombus in situ, or the vein may be seen as non-compressible. Duplex scanning combining the Doppler and B mode ultrasonography gives the anatomical features and functional information about the presence of clots or blood flow.
- Echocardiography may be done immediately by the bedside and can identify the thrombus rarely. Signs of right ventricular dilatation, right heart strain, tricuspid regurgitation, and inter ventricular septum bulging to the left side may be seen.
- Electrocardiography (ECG), rules out myocardial infarction, may show right ventricular strain pattern, right bundle branch block, right axis deviation and inverted T waves in V1 to V3 and S1Q3T3 pattern.
- Pulmonary venography can be done in selected patients, but is prone for complications such as iatrogenic dislodging, injury or allergy.
- Ventilation perfusion scan is a common screening technique. The probability estimates for PTE by evaluation of site and perfusion defects of lungs compared to ventilation. If normal, diagnosis is excluded.

- Impedance plethysmography to detect impaired venous emptying of lung is noninvasive, however, of limited value especially when DVT is asymptomatic, distal or nonocclusive.

TREATMENT

- Anticoagulation, thrombolysis, adjunctive measures, rarely surgery, and prophylaxis are the various modes of treatment.
- Anticoagulation therapy prevents further formation of clot. The patient's own fibrinolytic system dissolves the clot in due course of time.
- Thrombolysis treatment may be considered if there is a large thrombus causing hemodynamic instability.
- Surgical thrombectomy or venous interruption may be considered in rare circumstances when the above methods are considered not feasible options.
- Anticoagulation is initiated by unfractionated heparin (UFH) or low molecular weight heparin (LMWH), and then followed by oral anticoagulation. Initially, initiation of oral anticoagulants (OACs) may cause a procoagulant effect. Treatment with an oral coumarin derivative should start after 24–48 hours of adequate anticoagulation.
- International clinical practice guidelines for the treatment and prophylaxis of VTE in patients with cancer were issued by the American Society of Clinical Oncology (ASCO) in early 2013. Some of the recommendations are as follows:
  - For the initial treatment of established VTE, LMWH is recommended, and UFH can be also used
  - Thrombolysis may only be considered on a case-by-case basis
  - Vena cava filters (VCFs) may be considered if there is a contraindication to anticoagulation or PTE recurrence under optimal anticoagulation. They are not recommended for primary prophylaxis and even periodic reassessments of contraindications to anticoagulation are recommended
  - For the early maintenance and long-term treatment of established VTE, LMWH for a minimum of 3 months is preferred over vitamin K antagonists (VKAs). After 3–6 months, LMWH or VKA continuation should be based on individual evaluation of the benefits and risks, tolerability, patient preference and cancer activity
  - For the treatment of VTE recurrence in cancer patients receiving anticoagulation, there are three options:
    - Switch from VKA to LMWH when treated with VKA
    - Increase LMWH dose when treated with LMWH, and
    - VCF insertion
  - For the prophylaxis of postoperative VTE in surgical cancer patients, use of LMWH or low-dose UFH is recommended
  - Extended prophylaxis (4 weeks) after major laparotomy may be indicated in patients with a high risk of VTE and low risk of bleeding

- Use of LMWH for VTE prevention in cancer patients undergoing laparoscopic surgery may be recommended as for laparotomy
- Mechanical methods are not recommended as monotherapy except when pharmacologic methods are contraindicated
- In hospitalized patients with cancer and reduced mobility, prophylaxis with LMWH, UFH, or fondaparinux is recommended
- Routine prophylaxis is not recommended in patients receiving chemotherapy.
- Heparin given as a bolus of 80 mg/kg followed by an infusion of 18 mg/kg/h to titrate the activated partial thromboplastin time (aPTT) to 1.5–2 times the baseline is the first-line of treatment. It is worth mentioning that progression or recurrence of thromboembolism is 15 times more likely when a therapeutic aPTT is not achieved within the first 48 hours. Oral warfarin is started after adequate anticoagulation is established to maintain an international normalized ratio (INR) of 2.0–3.0 for a minimum of 3 months for the first episode.
- Alternatives to long-term oral anticoagulant therapy with warfarin are LMWH (considered if adequate means to administer it in patients with stable DVT) and newer oral anticoagulants (NOACs). While the initial trial results look encouraging, definitely more studies are required to determine their regular usage in long-term anticoagulation.

COMPLICATIONS

Development of post-thrombotic syndrome (postphlebitis syndrome) is a common complication characterized by pain and swelling of the lower limbs. Recurrent cellulitis and chronic venous insufficiency along with even ulceration may be seen.

Bleeding, especially with treatment with heparin or oral anticoagulation is common, and remains the most dreaded complication, especially in postsurgical patients.

Heparin-induced thrombocytopenia (HIT) is seen in patients within 5–10 days of treatment with heparin. It presents with a precipitous drop of platelet count.

Long-term treatment with UFH may cause osteopenia, while coumarin derivatives may cause skin necrosis.

Risk of secondary or recurrent thrombosis is 3–4%, and is higher in those with either proximal thrombi, or those with persistent risk factors. Long-term aspirin is shown to reduce the incidence of recurrent thrombosis as well as arterial thrombi.

PROPHYLAXIS

Prophylaxis reduces the risk of VTE. UFH prophylaxis should start 12 hours prior to surgery, or immediately after surgery, and should continue up to around 10 days.

Nonpharmacological prophylaxis includes pneumatic compression stockings, early ambulation and postdischarge prophylaxis with LMWH or NOACs.

CONCLUSION

Venous thromboembolism in the patient with gynecological cancers is an important condition causing much mortality and morbidity. Identifying the at risk patients, adequate prophylactic measures, smart recognition at an early stage of the disease, postdischarge prophylaxis, and long-term treatment with anticoagulants reduce the incidence and morbidity/mortality of the dreaded condition.

Chapter 6

Para-Aortic Lymphadenectomy in Gynecologic Malignancies

Somashekhar SP

Refer to my Operative video of the same for detailed steps and technique along with this:

INDICATIONS

1. Carcinoma ovary—as part of proper and complete staging surgery in early ovarian cancer
2. Carcinoma ovary—in stage III ovarian surgery with bulky para-aortic lymph nodes after optimal cytoreduction
3. Carcinoma endometrium—high-risk carcinoma endometrium as staging surgery.

INCISION

1. Midline laparotomy with supraumbilical extension—transperitoneal approach
2. Bilateral flank incision J-shaped—retroperitoneal approach
3. Laparoscopic retroperitoneal approach.

BOUNDARIES OF PARA-AORTIC LYMPHADENECTOMY

- Upper extent: Both renal veins
- Right: Right lateral border of inferior vena cava (IVC)
- Left: Left lateral border of aorta
- Inferiorly: Division of aorta into common Iliac
- Posteriorly: Anterior spinal ligament.

Note: The most important nodes in para-aortic dissection are the nodes between renal veins and inferior mesenteric artery.

On the right side: Most important node is paracaval nodes at the level of joining of ovarian vein to IVC, via infundibulopelvic ligament—nodes and lymphatics lie primarily in the vena caval fat bed.

On the left side: Most important node is para-aortic nodes at the fork of left renal vein, and left lateral border of aorta via left ovarian vein draining to left renal vein—nodes and lymphatics lie posterior to aorta.

Techniques

1. Lateral peritoneal incision approach, mobilizing colon—Cattell-Braasch maneuver—mobilizing right colon medially and left colon medially
2. Midline peritoneal incision approach—incising peritoneum over common iliac arteries and aorta.

Operative Steps

- Inverted J-shaped incision is placed along right line of Toldt, right to the ascending colon and continuing upward about 4 cm short of hepatic flexure of colon and inferiorly the inverted J extending below and to the left of cecum—Cattell-Braasch maneuver.
- The entire right colon along with mesentery of small bowel is mobilized toward midline—this is avascular plane and gives immediate and good access to retroperitoneum, IVC and aorta easily. The mobilization from right to left across midline until third part of duodenum and both renal veins are exposed (T12-L1 junction).
- Whole of small bowel is wrapped in saline soaked towel and swung upward to the chest of the patient.
- Ureter will always go with the roof of this peritoneum and needs to be separated carefully and pushed to the right side along with its mesentery and twigs of blood supply.
- Now hold the tied ends of right ovarian vessels and follow and trace them upward, until they open to IVC on right side and on the left side until they open to left renal vein, clamp the same at the level of termination and tie and cut them—this is the road map to the retroperitoneal lymph nodes and exposure to renal veins.
- Retract the duodenum, and start systematic para-aortic and paracaval lymphadenectomy. Boundaries are renal veins above, division of aorta below and right to IVC and left of aorta.
- Systematic dissection encompassing all the fat, lymphatics and lymph nodes, of right paracaval, precaval, retrocaval, interaortocaval, preaortic, left para-aortic, retroaortic lymph nodal tissues are removed and labeled and sent for histopathological examination (HPE).
- Dissection can be done with diathermy, blunt tip in spray mode, setting of 36 or alternately using Metzenbaum sharp scissors. Special attention must be given to consistent tributaries joining IVC about 2–4 cm above the division to common iliac vein and lumbar vein joining IVC and renal veins

from posteriorly. They must be specifically sought, identified and ligated/clipped to prevent catastrophic bleeding. Venous bleeding is low pressure but high volume, while arterial bleeding would be high pressure, but low volume. If any bleeding occurs from IVC, just proximal pressure with finger and identification of rent in decompressed veins and suture ligation will promptly control the same.

- Once the preaortic nodal dissection reaches inferior mesenteric artery (L2 level) special attention has to be paid in identifying and preserving inferior mesenteric plexus of sympathetic nerves along with inferior mesenteric artery which, go on to become hypogastric plexus of nerves. This will help in early recovery of bowel function.
- With sharp scissor dissection, left renal veins are identified and especially the nodes in the fork of aorta, left renal veins are removed. Now the assistant retracts both the IVC and aorta laterally and the interaortocaval nodal tissue with nodes is removed, until anterior spinal ligament is exposed. This is a glistening tough longitudinal ligament, exposure of which shows the completeness of the dissection. With the assistant retracting and swing IVC and aorta toward midline, the retrocaval and retroaortic nodes are dissected and removed.
- Once systematic lymphadenectomy is done, thorough hemostasis is achieved and the mobilized colon and bowel to position, no fixation or reperitonealization is required. No need to keep drains either.
- I prefer doing the entire surgery with spray mode coagulation diathermy settings of 36 without use of clips.
- After good irrigation and saline wash, abdomen is closed in monolayer with all interrupted Prolene no. 1 suture, near-far suture technique. I prefer grossing and labeling the lymph nodes personally at the end of procedure before sending the specimen for HPE.

Chapter 7

Diaphragm Stripping and Resection in Ovarian Cancer

Somashekhar SP

Refer to my Operative video of the same for detailed steps and technique along with this.

INDICATIONS

1. In stage-III, ovarian cancer as part of optimal cytoreduction after achieving complete resection of pelvic and peritoneal disease
2. Following neoadjuvant chemotherapy as part of interval debluking, in right upper abdomen diaphragm disease
3. In recurrent disease in right upper abdomen, diaphragm disease as part of secondary debulking after disease-free survival (DFS) of over 1–2 years.

INCISION

- Midline laparotmy incision reaching up to xiphisternum
- Bilateral subcostal self-retaining retractors (Kelly's or Mayo-Brown or Omni retractor) application would be very useful in diaphragm stripping or resection.

PROCEDURE

- First and foremost important step in diaphragm stripping or resection is mobilization of liver and cutting all its ligamentous attachment and swinging and retraction liver to left and to midline, towards main laparotomy incision and identifying inferior vena cava (IVC) and right hepatic vein.
- First clamp, cut falciform ligament, trace its lower border, which continues as ligament of teres up to the diaphragm. Here it divides into two leaves in triangular manner, trace and cut the same with diatheramy

up to T8 level of diaphragm near the central tendon of diaphragm. This leads to opening in diaphragm where IVC enters. Using Metzenbaum scissors, sharp dissection is done and IVC and right hepatic veins are identified and guarded.

- Now Left triangular, right triangular ligaments are cut and superior, and inferior coronory ligaments are mobilized and the loose peritoneal attachments of liver to Morison's pouch and prerenal fascia are all mobilized. Now liver hangs only by IVC and hepatic veins and it can easily be turned to main wound and retracted, and entire retrohepatic portion of IVC is under vision.

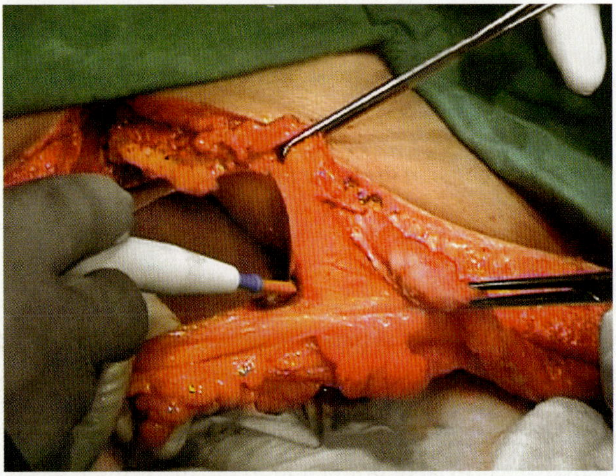

Fig. 1: Falciform ligament clamped and cut as part of liver mobilization. (*Courtesy:* Dr Somashekhar SP)

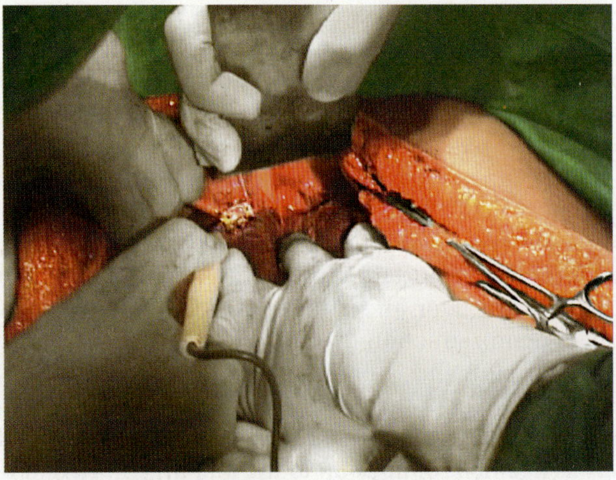

Fig. 2: Cutting triangular ligaments–Mobilization of liver. (*Courtesy:* Dr Somashekhar SP)

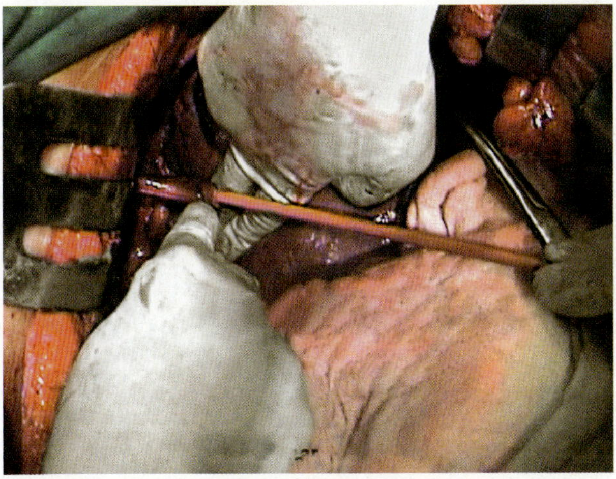

Fig. 3: Evacuation of pneumothorax using red rubber catheter with low pressure suction–avoids ICD placement.
(*Courtesy:* Dr Somashekhar SP)

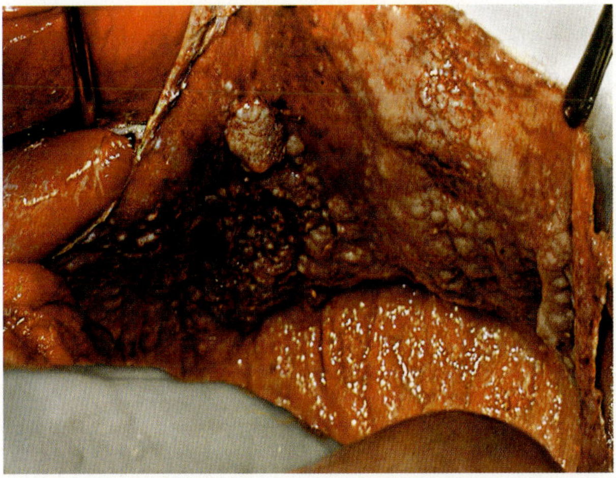

Fig. 4: Bulky diaphragm nodules cytoreduced by stripping.
(*Courtesy:* Dr Somashekhar SP)

- Now the whole of diaphragm is exposed and seen like a mat completely under vision. Application of self-retaining costal retractors now will aid the stripping and resection very easy now.
- Now stripping of diaphragm peritoneal surface is started from lower border of costal arch. Initially using diathermy, the entire border of peritoneum to be stripped is marked first from lower border of costal arch to peritoneal reflection up to infrahepatic portion near Morison's pouch and laterally up to paracolic gutter and medially up to midline near central tendon

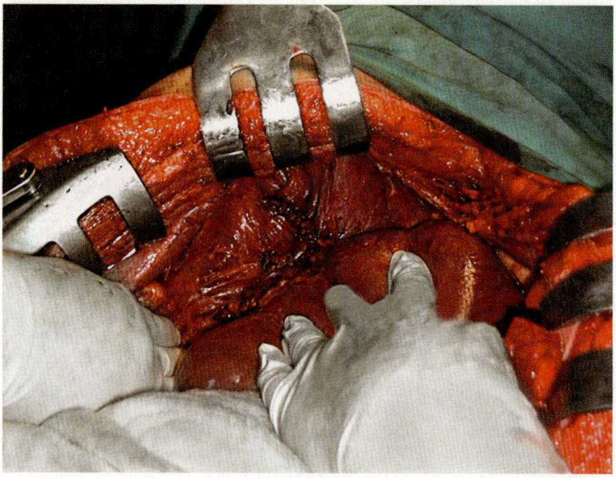

Fig. 5: Prolene sutured diaphragm after full thickness resection of up to 30% of diaphragm–No ICD placed.
(*Courtesy:* Dr Somashekhar SP)

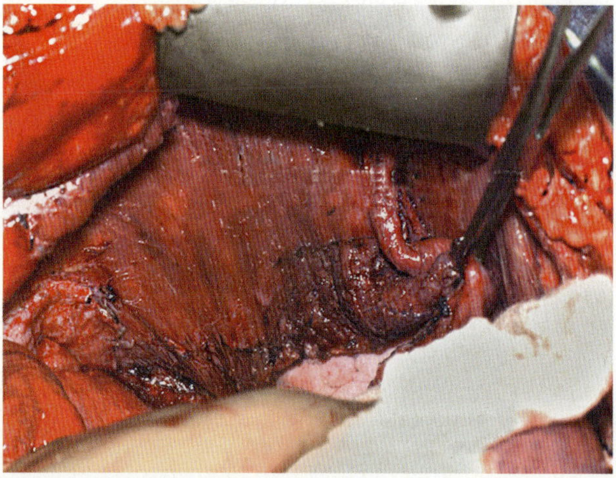

Fig. 6: Stripped diaphragm with superfical fibers of muscle—but intact pleura.
(*Courtesy:* Dr Somashekhar SP)

of diaphragm on which beating heart rests and inferiorly up to coronary ligament over liver, which is the boundary of bare area of liver.

- Stripping of diaphragm peritoneum can be done by combination of sharp dissection using diathermy or Metzenbaum scissors or blunt dissection using combination of double swab or single swab technique.
- I personally prefer using spray mode of coagulation diathermy setting No. 36 with combination of double swab technique giving traction and counter traction for entire stripping. Using this technique, the entire diaphragm

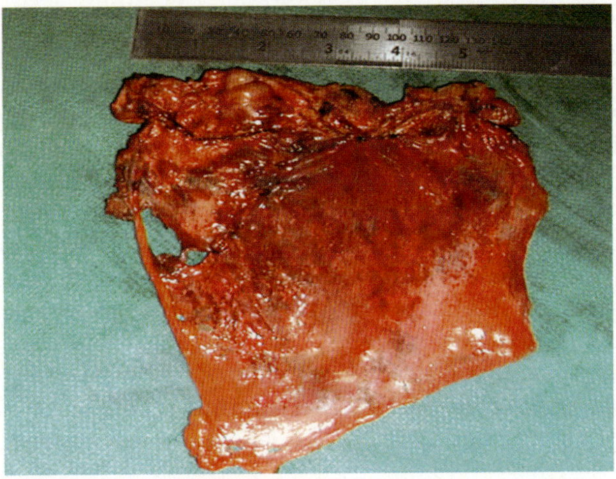

Fig. 7: Specimen of stripped and resected diaphragm with nodules in pleura. (*Courtesy:* Dr Somashekhar SP)

peritoneum with all nodules and bulky disease. It can easily be stripped as single piece like a matt. It is stripped up to the superior coronary ligament of liver forming the superior boundary of bare area of liver. This preserves the diaphragm muscle fibers completely untouched and intact.

- Special attention has to be given to identify and preserve inferior phrenic vessels, which run parallel to the costal arch posteriorly at the level of T12 from aorta.
- The diaphragm stripping is combined with diaphragm resection when and where the disease invades diaphragm musculature fullness. The part of this needs to be resected.
- Once the stripping reaches the point of invasion of musculature, resection starts. Using diathermy the full thickness of muscle is cut and once a rent is created gaining access to right pleural cavity, lower border of right lung is visualized and adhesions released, and lung is retracted and guarded. Now keeping finger inside the pleural cavity the entire part of diaphragm invaded along with full-thickness pleura attached to superior surface of diaphragm is resected using diathermy as single piece keeping it attached to the stripped part of diaphragm *(Please refer to my operative video for this detailed step)*
- When the part is invading is close or adherent to glisson capsule of liver, change the coagulation mode of spray mode of diathermy setting from 36 to 100 and slowly using the diathermy cut close to glisson capsule or liver parenchyma and resect the diseased diaphragm with part of capsule and parenchyma of liver in perfect hemostatic way. Previous orientation and exposure of IVC and right hepatic veins help this step easily.
- Resected diaphragm is sutured back. Up to about 30% of defect can easily be sutured primarily, alternately if the defect is big, Marlex mesh or Gortex patch is used. Suturing can be done in two layers using polydioxanone

(PDS), continuous and prolene interrupted or alternatively using prolene as single layer continuous suturing technique. While resecting and suturing diaphragm, special attention should be payed towards orientation of phrenic nerve and avoid cutting or entrapping the same in sutures.

- Most of the cases does not require placement of intercostal drainage tube (ICD). The suturing of diaphragm is continued to the end and a small red rubber tube catheter is inserted via the rent inside the pleural cavity and, low pressure continuous suction is applied and all the liquid and air in pleural cavity is sucked out before tightening the purse string suture at the end of suturing. This in most of cases prevents pneumothorax and avoids placement of ICD tube.
- No need to place drainage tube and abdomen is closed using prolene No. 1 monolayer all interrupted near-far suturing technique.
- Resected and stripped specimen is oriented and sent for HPE.

Chapter 8

Gyne-Oncology Surgery: Metaplastic Thoughts from Benign to Malignant

Sabhyata Gupta, Shradha Chaudhari

Metaplasia is a change happening at a cellular level, pushing a normal tissue through a journey associated with a variable outcome. In the last few decades, the field of Gyne-Oncology surgery has witnessed a paradigmatic and metaplastic change with a shift towards new technology, fertility preservation and a less radical surgical approach.

In this metaplastic journey, the field of Gyne-Oncology has witnessed a redefining moment with the introduction of robotic technology to gynecological cancers. Food and Drug Administration (US FDA or FDA) has approved the use of da Vinci robotic surgical system for its application in gynecology in 2005. Since then, it has gained acceptance rapidly and has now emerged as a standard of care worldwide for minimally invasive surgery for carcinoma endometrium and carcinoma cervix. The standard laparoscopic route is technically more difficult to adopt and only a small subset of surgeons can perform oncological surgery using standard laparoscopy. Robotic technology has made minimally invasive surgery possible for a larger platform of surgeons. The minimally invasive route follows all oncological principles of surgery, takes similar operative time as compared to open route and has lesser blood loss. The lymph node retrieval rate is also comparable to the earlier standard laparotomy. The faster healing in the postoperative period renders the patient fit, quickly for adjuvant radiation or chemotherapy.

A paradigm shift has already happened in minimally invasive surgery. Intuitive surgical, the company manufacturing da Vinci surgical robots has recently received FDA approval for the expanded indication of the company's Firefly system to visualize blood vasculature in real time. Indocyanine green (ICG) dye is injected into the bloodstream which naturally sticks to the albumin. When a 803 nm wavelength laser illuminates the surgical scene, the dye is excited and glows, showing the path of vessels thus helping the surgeon to identify these vessels. ICG can also be injected into the cervix or endometrium to detect the sentinel node during the surgical staging of carcinoma endometrium. The detection rate of sentinel node is higher with ICG as compared to methylene blue dye or technetium-99m colloid. Some of the centers in the west are using a frozen section on sentinel node to decide the extent of pelvic and para-aortic lymph node dissection in the staging of carcinoma endometrium; this reduces the morbidity associated with lymphadenectomy. Similarly, the detection of sentinel nodes using ICG dye is now possible in newer versions of the systems used in laparoscopic surgery. Thus, application of sentinel node mapping is extended to laparoscopic route as well.

A variety of less known indications like groin node dissection for carcinoma vulva can also be operated upon by using robotics. In fertility-sparing surgery for carcinoma cervix, robotic trachelectomy and pelvic lymphadenectomy are now emerging to be feasible, and studies have reported this surgery even in very young girls. There are also a few reports of robotic surgery for early-stage ovarian cancer. However, laparotomy remains standard of care for proven ovarian malignancies. Port site metastasis rates are significantly higher in minimally invasive surgery performed in ovarian cancer.

Standard laparoscopic surgery is still the preferred mode of surgery for complex adnexal masses. To understand what the surgeon will be dealing with, a preoperative workup is necessary. Magnetic resonance imaging (MRI) is the most superior radiological imaging to understand the nature of the ovarian cyst and to look for suspicious malignancy. The associated tumor markers like CA 125, HE4, beta-HCG, AFP, estradiol and inhibin B must be done depending on the nature of the cyst on imaging. The surgeon must follow all oncological principles of surgery including prevention of accidental rupture of the ovarian cyst and spill of its contents in the abdominal cavity by using endobag and preventive steps for port site metastasis like thorough lavage of the abdominal ports prior to closure. In case of suspected malignancy, the intraoperative frozen section must be done. If the frozen section is positive, then complete surgical staging must be done in the same sitting. Thus, it is not mandatory to perform laparotomy for all complex ovarian masses.

After the revolution in the surgical technique, the most recent advancement has been an increasing focus on fertility preservation in cancers. With the coining of the new term 'oncofertility', it is clear that fertility preservation and oncology must go hand in hand.

In all stage IA ovarian cancers and borderline ovarian cancers, where fertility is desired, fertility preservation surgery can be performed and conservation of the contralateral ovary and uterus allows for the women to plan future pregnancy once surgery, radiation and chemotherapy is complete. Few centers have reported laparoscopic and robotic route of surgery for early-stage IA ovarian cancers.

In women desirous of childbearing and having been diagnosed with newly detected well differentiated endometrioid carcinoma endometrium with disease limited to endometrium, high dose progestin therapy can be administered. Follow up with three-monthly endometrial biopsies can either show regression or persistence of disease. Therapy can be used for a period of 12 months to look for a desired response in the change from malignant to benign on endometrial biopsy. Once proven benign, the patient can plan for natural conception or assisted reproduction. Once her childbearing is complete, she needs to undergo complete surgery for the cancer. Apart from a high dose of oral progesterone (like megestrol acetate or medroxyprogesterone acetate), studies have reported the use of levonorgestrel-releasing intrauterine device to treat early stage endometrial cancer. However, patients opting for fertility-preserving treatment for early-stage carcinoma endometrium must be adequately counseled that this is not standard of care and that complete surgery is mandatory once childbearing is complete or in case of failure of progestin therapy.

Fertility preservation surgery can also be performed in early stages of carcinoma cervix. Conization of the cervix was described many years back. Traditionally, it was performed with cold knife. Now loop electrosurgical excision procedure (LEEP) is also an acceptable method to perform conization provided adequate surgical margins and proper orientation of the cone are obtained. Trachelectomy (simple/radical with pelvic lymphadenectomy) can be performed in early stage 1 cervical cancers. Approaches include abdominal route, vaginal route, laparoscopy and the most recent being a robotic route.

Apart from surgical technique and fertility preservation, another major change in surgery in the field of Gyne-Oncology is revolutionized surgical armamentarium. Newer instruments made surgery both easier and safer. Vessel-sealing devices and cutting devices like the LigaSure, Harmonic Ace, EnSeal and PG Gyrus are available. They are more effective in sealing vessels and at the same time have inbuilt safety features. Collateral thermal damage with these instruments is minimal as compared to standard bipolar and monopolar cautery. These devices are also manufactured in various sizes and shapes suitable for the open route of surgery or laparoscopic route. Instruments are also designed for single port laparoscopic and robotic surgery.

Gone are the days of aggressive and extensive dissection for surgery in gynecological cancers. Trends in Gyne-Oncology surgery are all metamorphosed to make cancer surgery safe, fast, less invasive and bring the patient back to a normal healthy condition as soon as feasible without compromising the oncological outcome. The patient's overall quality of life, disease-free interval and survival rates have improved significantly. The future of Gyne-Oncology will bring in more such developments to make life with cancer less challenging and life after cancer treatment healthy and happy. Thus metaplasia from benign to malignant will be reversed. The malignant effect of gynecological cancer will reduce, thus making the disease appear 'benign.'

Chapter 9

Peritonectomy in Ovarian Malignancy

Brig Manash Biswas

INTRODUCTION

Epithelial ovarian cancer comprises 90% of all ovarian cancers. Like most other epithelial tumors, epithelial ovarian cancer spreads initially by direct extension into adjacent organs, especially the fallopian tubes, uterus, and contralateral adnexa, and, occasionally, the rectum, bladder, and pelvic sidewall are also invaded.[1] After direct extension, epithelial ovarian cancer most frequently disseminates via the transcelomic route, with about 70% of patients having peritoneal metastases at staging laparotomy. Hematogenous metastases are almost never present at diagnosis.[1]

Transcelomic metastases are often associated with the formation of malignant ascites, resulting in raised intra-abdominal pressure and consequent abdominal distention and discomfort, early satiety leading to dietary deficiency, impaired circulation of blood and lymphatic vessels, and respiratory embarrassment secondary to diaphragmatic splinting.[2] Although the cause of ovarian cancer remains mostly unknown, most epithelial ovarian carcinomas have been suggested to arise from the ovarian surface epithelium, which has its embryonic origins in the celomic mesothelium.[3] The celomic mesothelium can evolve into serous (tubal), endometrioid (endometrium), and mucinous (cervix) epithelia of the female genital tract, and the ovarian surface epithelium is a specialized celomic mesothelial layer of flat to cuboidal cells that covers and protects the ovary.[4]

THE TRANSCELOMIC JOURNEY

Mechanisms of Transcelomic Metastasis in Ovarian Cancer (Fig. 1)

Step 1: Epithelial ovarian cancer cell (green) detaches after altered gene expression.

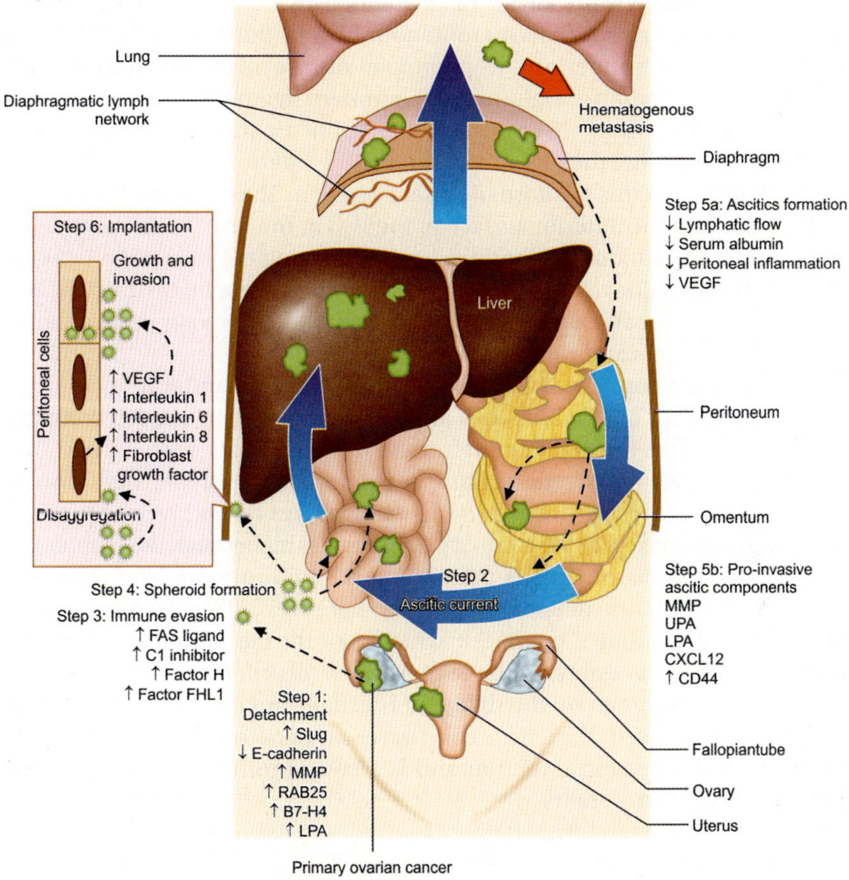

Fig. 1: Mechanisms of transcelomic metastasis in ovarian cancer.
(B7-H4=Immune co-stimulatory protein B7-H4; CXCL12=ligand of chemokine (CXC motif) receptor 4 (CXCR4); FHL1=factor H-like protein 1; LPA=lysophosphatidic acid.)
Source: Mechanisms of transcoelomic metastasis in ovarian cancer. Lancet Oncol. 2006;7:925-34.

Step 2: Peritoneal or ascitic current (blue arrows) facilitates peritoneal, lymphatic, and hematogenous metastasis.

Step 3: Immune evasion by complement inhibition and secretion of FAS ligand.

Step 4: Spheroid formation.

Step 5: Ascetic components stimulate further metastatic progression.

Step 6: Peritoneal activation and implantation.

Anatomy

Primary anatomic considerations for diaphragm surgery include the relevant hepatic attachments and the underlying central vasculature. The anterior hepatic attachment is the falciform ligament, which attaches the liver to the anterior abdominal wall in its membranous hepatic portion. As the falciform ligament continues superiorly, its peritoneal surface divides laterally on each side to form the anterior right and left coronary ligaments. These coronary ligaments reflect off the liver capsule and delineate the posterior extent of peritoneum covering the diaphragm above. The inferior vena cava (IVC) lies to the right side of this falciform ligament division. The right and left hepatic veins drain into the anterior surface of the IVC at the level of this peritoneal reflection, and caution is essential when performing the dissection to avoid injury to these major vessels. In addition, the lateral branches of the right and left inferior phrenic artery and vein may be encountered laterally in the anterior coronary ligaments and can be divided as required.[5]

The anterior coronary ligaments continue laterally and inferiorly along the posterior liver edge where they join the posterior right and left coronary ligaments to form the right and left triangular ligaments, respectively. The right triangular ligament reflects from the liver to the diaphragm, right kidney, and right adrenal gland. The left triangular ligament reflects primarily to the diaphragm; the posterior left coronary ligament lies higher than the esophageal hiatus, and the esophagus is generally not encountered. The coronary ligaments on each side delineate the larger "bare area" of the liver on the right and a smaller "bare area" on the left, which underlie the central tendon of the diaphragm. The right phrenic nerve penetrates this central tendon lateral to the vena caval foramen on the right and is usually not encountered until the "bare area" is exposed. The left phrenic nerve may penetrate the left diaphragm muscle above the central tendon and is a consideration during left-sided anterior diaphragm surgery.

Equipment Needed

Fixed retractor system with or without a Balfour retractor; electrocautery; Allis clamps; long Metzenbaum scissors; long forceps; long Mixter clamp; headlamp; argon beam coagulator set at 70–90 W.

Procedure

The first and an important step is of achieving adequate liver mobilization. Once an exploratory laparotomy has been performed and the presence of bulky diaphragm disease confirmed on one or both hemidiaphragms, the midline incision is extended to the xiphoid process (Fig. 2). Due to the depth and irregular contours of the subphrenic space, an operating headlamp facilitates illumination and a fixed retractor system is essential (Fig. 3). The retractor should be set at an adequate height to retract the costal margins superolaterally. The lateral blades of a Balfour retractor can be used to separate the incision laterally in the midline. Retractor blade selection is determined by patient features— deeper blades utilized for patients with thicker subcutaneous adipose tissue, and blades placed more medially for patients with a deeper chest cavity.

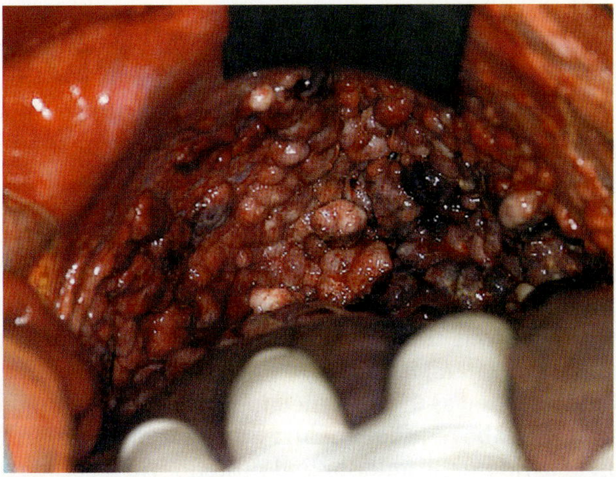

Fig. 2: Large-volume diaphragm disease. With the surgeon's left hand applying downward traction to the right hepatic lobe, the full extent of large-volume diaphragm disease is appreciated.

Source: Atlas of Procedures in Gynecologic Oncology, Levine, Barakat, and Hoskins.

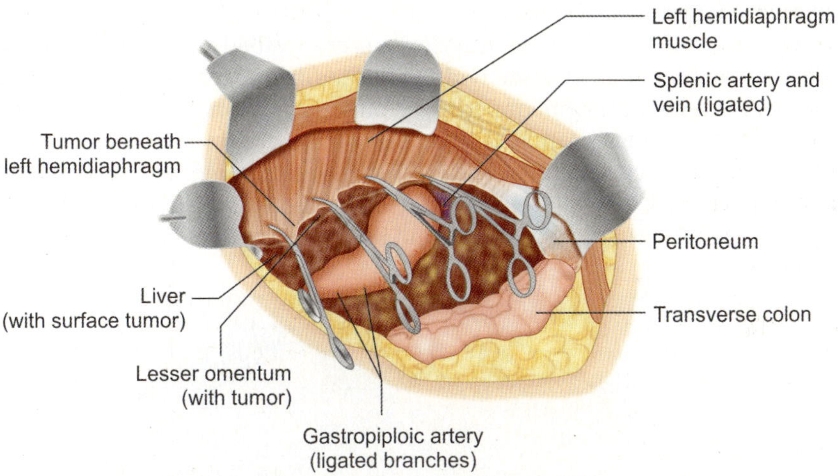

Fig. 3: Left subphrenic peritonectomy.

Source: PH Sugarbaker/Surg Oncol Clin N Am 12 (2003).

The extent of liver mobilization required depends on the distribution of tumor involving the hemidiaphragm. Large volume disease is common on the right side.

Tumor involvement on the left diaphragm is more easily resected without fully mobilizing the liver, although in certain cases splenectomy may be necessary to clear the metastatic deposits.

The infrahepatic edge of the falciform ligament containing the ligamentum teres is grasped between two Kelly clamps, divided, and ligated. The suture on the lower edge is left long enough to aid with downward traction of the liver and remaining falciform ligament. Once the ligamentum teres is divided, the membranous portion of the falciform ligament is incised superiorly with the cautery, freeing the hepatic attachment to the anterior abdominal wall. A combination of gentle downward pressure on the liver with a moist laparotomy sponge and downward tension on the falciform ligament suture facilitates this medial dissection. As the superior edge of the liver is approached, the falciform ligament splays laterally on each side to become continuous with the anterior right and left coronary ligaments. The anterior right coronary ligament is divided with the awareness that the distal right hepatic vein and IVC lie just beneath the plane of dissection. Peritoneal dissection is then continued laterally along the anterior right coronary ligament until limited by visualization, and lateral branches of the inferior phrenic artery and vein are clipped or cauterized as they are encountered (Fig. 4). The right triangular ligament is divided above the renal and adrenal reflection on the right. A combination of dividing the anterior and posterior right coronary ligaments will allow the right hepatic lobe to be mobilized medially until the previous dissection along the anterior right coronary ligament can be joined. We have outlined here the steps for freeing the hepatic attachments, but the specific sequence of steps will vary from patient to patient based on the tumor distribution and ease of exposure.

The extent of diaphragm peritonectomy is determined by the distribution of the tumor implants, and the method can be modified accordingly. To perform a full right sided diaphragmatic peritonectomy, the peritoneum on the anterior edge of the diaphragm is incised along the costal margin using either cautery or Metzenbaum scissors. This anterior free edge is grasped with several Allis or Mixter clamps, which are then retracted inferiorly to visualize the line of attachment between the diaphragm and its overlying peritoneum. The plane

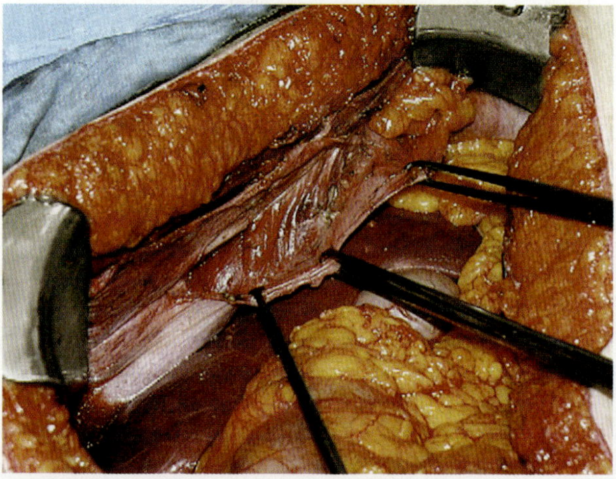

Fig. 4: Peritoneal incision. The peritoneum on the anterior edge of the right hemi-diaphragm is incised along the costal margin, grasped with several Allis clamps, and the line of attachment between the diaphragm muscle and overlying peritoneum identified.

Source: Atlas of Procedures in Gynecologic Oncology. Levine, Barakat, and Hoskins.

between is developed with a combination of blunt and sharp dissection as determined by the patient's tissue laxity and/or peritoneal adherence. The upward retraction of the costal margin allows the operating surgeon to provide downward traction on the peritoneum with one hand and perform the dissection with the other so that the tension and subsequent depth of dissection along the thin diaphragm muscle can be controlled. The anesthesiologist is notified on handling of the liver especially on its medial rotation, as increase in vagal tone can precipitate transient bradycardia and hypotension. The specimen can be removed en bloc, if feasible, but segmental resection may be necessary to improve exposure.

The main problems for the peritonectomy relate to diaphragm penetration. Small blood vessels, most often branches from the inferior phrenic artery and vein, can be clipped or coagulated. Hemostasis during diaphragm peritonectomy is most easily achieved with the argon beam coagulator. Since the right phrenic nerve and IVC pass through foramina in the liver "bare area", they are outside the plane of dissection during diaphragm peritonectomy. Even when the peritoneal surface is studded with tumor implants, it can usually be cleanly separated from the underlying musculature. Tumor implants that are securely fixed to the diaphragm muscle are suspicious for full-thickness diaphragm involvement, and diaphragm resection should be considered.

Smaller areas of full thickness involvement can be tented downwards away from the pleura and Endo GIA stapled, simultaneously resecting the diseased area and restoring the diaphragmatic continuity.

After the peritonectomy has been completed, a "bubble test" is performed to identify small diaphragm penetration sites (Fig. 5).[5] The patient is placed in shallow Trendelenburg, and the ipsilateral upper quadrant filled with saline.

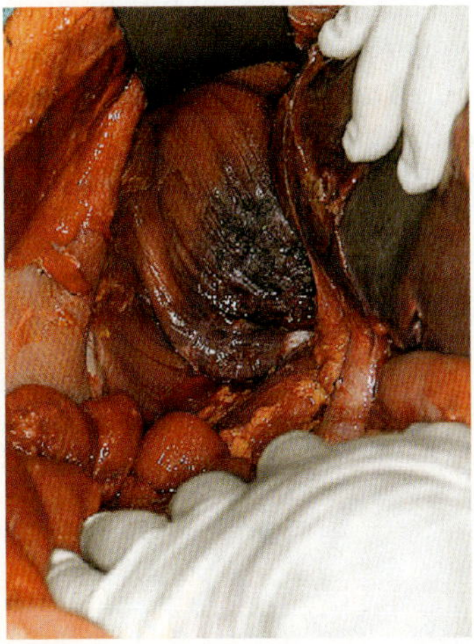

Fig. 5: Peritonectomy completed. With the peritonectomy completed, the diaphragm musculature can be viewed entirely. The liver has been fully mobilized and retracted medially, allowing the inferior vena cava to be visualized beneath the surgeon's left index finger as it travels behind the liver.

Source: Atlas of Procedures in Gynecologic Oncology. Levine, Barakat, and Hoskins.

Air bubbles on inspiration will indicate whether a perforation has occurred. These defects are closed primarily to prevent the sequelae of an untreated pneumothorax. Small visible defects can be closed in the following fashion. A purse-string suture is placed widely around the hole and a 14 French feeding tube is passed through the hole into the pleural cavity. The anesthesiologist is asked to give the patient a maximal inspiration, suction may be applied to the catheter, and the catheter is pulled as the purse-string suture is tied down. Larger defects can be closed with a series of either interrupted horizontal mattress or figure-of-eight permanent sutures.

All patients undergoing diaphragm surgery should have a chest radiograph in the post-operative care unit.[6] Significant pneumothorax is managed with chest tube placement. The majority of patients develop an ipsilateral postoperative pleural effusion, and few will require subsequent pleural drainage. Patients are followed up with daily postoperative chest radiographs until the effusion size stabilizes. Complications, such as hemothorax, are rare and can usually be avoided with close attention to hemostasis during diaphragm resection.

RATIONALE FOR PERITONECTOMY PROCEDURES

If a surgeon elects to manage patients with primary surgery in ovarian malignancies, additional knowledge concerning cancer dissemination on peritoneal surfaces and numerous refinements of his or her technical skills are required. Peritonectomy procedures are necessary if one is to successfully treat ovarian malignancies with optimal cytoreduction in many instances (Fig. 6). Peritonectomy procedures are used in the areas of visible cancer progression in an attempt to leave the patient with only microscopic residual disease. In addition to stripping of peritoneal surfaces, small tumor nodules are removed using electroevaporation. Involvement of visceral peritoneum frequently requires resection of a portion of the stomach, small intestine, or colorectum. Usually a complete pelvic peritonectomy involves stripping of the abdominal sidewalls, the peritoneum overlying the bladder, the cul-de-sac, and the rectosigmoid colon.

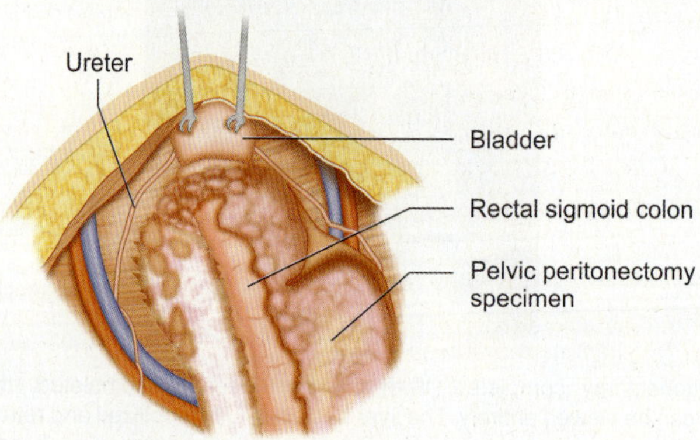

Fig. 6: Stripping the visceral peritoneum from the surface of the bladder.
Source: PH Sugarbaker. Surg Oncol Clin N Am. 12 (2003).

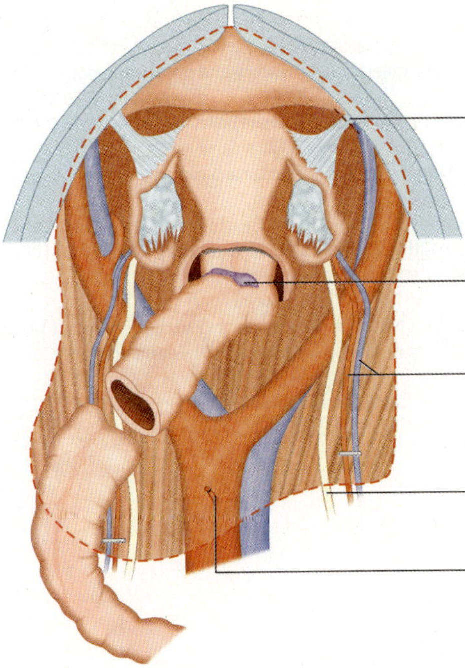

Fig. 7: Limits of the complete pelvic peritonectomy.
Source: PH Sugarbaker. Surg Oncol Clin N Am 12. (2003).

The surgical procedure would thereafter be completed by securing the vaginal vault, mobilizing the left colon and a colorectal anastomosis.

PROCEDURAL COMPLICATIONS

Perhaps the most difficult peritonectomy is the lesser omentectomy with stripping of the omental bursa.[7] Vital structures here are of great density and mistakes in dissection can lead to life-endangering hemorrhage or sever damage to the liver (Fig. 7). The left hepatic artery is the most commonly traumatized vessel. Also, loss of the left gastric artery may result in the need for total gastrectomy. Ligation of the left gastric vein may cause gastric portal hypertension when all other venous drainage of the stomach is removed by dissection around this organ. The left hepatic vein or left inferior phrenic vein are thin-walled, and may be damaged inadvertently by sudden and unpredictable diaphragmatic contractions stimulated by electrosurgical dissection near the crus of the right hemidiaphragm.

Multiple peritonectomy procedures are necessary if one is aiming for maximal surgical effort to successfully treat peritoneal dissemination of ovarian malignancies. It is unusual for all of these procedures to be needed for a single patient. If low-volume disease is being treated, the pelvic peritonectomy may be the most frequently performed procedure.

REFERENCES

1. Amadori D, Sansoni E, Amadori A. Ovarian cancer: natural history and metastatic pattern. Front Biosci. 1997;2:g8-10.
2. Tan DSP, Agarwal R, Kaye SB. Mechanisms of transcoelomic metastasis in ovarian cancer. Lancet Oncol. 2006;7(11):925-34.
3. Auersperg N, Wong AS, Choi KC, et al. Ovarian surface epithelium: biology, endocrinology, and pathology. Endocr Rev. 2001;22(2):255-88.
4. Crum CP. The female genital tract (chapter 22). In Kumar V, Fausto N, Abbas A, eds. Robbins and Cotran's Pathologic basis of disease. 7th edn. Philadelphia: Saunders, 2004:1059-118.
5. Eisenhauer EL, Chi DS. Liver mobilization and diaphragm peritonectomy/resection. Gynecol Oncol. 2007;104: S25-8.
6. Eisenhauer EL, D'Angelica MI, Abu-Rustum NR, et al. Incidence and management of pleural effusions after diaphragm peritonectomy or resection for advanced müllerian cancer. Gynecol Oncol. 2006;103(3):871-7.
7. Sugarbaker PH. Peritonectomy procedures. Surg Oncol Clin N Am. 2003;12(3):703-27.

Chapter 10

Postoperative Follow-Up after Gynecological Cancers: The Necessary Guidelines

Rupinder Sekhon, Jiten Jaipuria

INTRODUCTION

Gynecological cancers remain one of the most common cancers affecting Indian women with cervical, endometrial and ovarian cancers, constituting the majority. Unfortunately, majority of women in India present at an advanced stage due to various socioeconomic reasons which puts them at significant risk of recurrence, following initial definitive management. Also, since the majority of gynecological neoplasms present in the 4th and 5th decades, clinicians must observe diligence during post-treatment follow-up as there are decades of potential life spans at risk if an early recurrence is missed. Surprisingly, evidence-based follow-up protocols are lacking for most gynecological cancers and presently, most recommendations by international societies and cancer working groups are based on expert consensus and clinical best practices heavily influenced by other solid malignancies. Certain aspects of post-treatment surveillance remain common to all malignancies such as:

- *Patient education*: Educating patients about symptoms of recurrence is the cornerstone of a successful surveillance program as it elicits patient's cooperation and prevents unfortunate losses to follow-up. It also allows stakeholders to detect recurrences earlier than what a fixed follow-up schedule would have allowed. It's also considered a clinical best practice to teach patients periodic self-examination wherever, nature of malignancy allows (for e.g., vulvar cancer).
- *Counseling about treatment outcomes:* Patients should also be counseled about the nature of long-term and late-occurring complications which go a long way in allaying anxiety of confusing new onset symptoms with recurrence.
- *Nutritional counseling:* It is a frequently neglected aspect of follow-up and many patients continue to suffer from undernutrition by virtue of ill effects of recurrent disease (cancer-related cachexia) or original treatment whether it be surgical (gastrointestinal stomas and urinary conduits) or medical

(radiotherapy and chemotherapy with attendant blunted appetite and side effects such as diarrhea and proctitis).

- *Lifestyle advise:* Lifestyle advise such as promoting exercise, smoking cessation and reducing obesity have been shown to have beneficial effects in primary prevention of many cancers (including gynecological). Though there is no direct evidence of its beneficial effect in secondary prevention (trying to detect a disease early and prevent it from getting worse) and tertiary prevention (improve quality of life and reduce symptoms of an existing disease) of malignancies yet, it definitely has a beneficial effect in prolonging life in general.
- *Sexual health*: Princeton III Consensus Conference concluded that there is an increasing evidence in favor of sexual health as a surrogate marker for overall and cardiovascular health status among females.[1] Sexual rehabilitation after mutilating gynecologic surgeries can be problematic. However, a multidisciplinary approach with involvement of both partners in a relationship can be rewarding in many apparently difficult circumstances.

Also, since majority of the recurrences (more than 75%) for gynecological malignancies occur in the first 2 years, National Comprehensive Cancer Network (NCCN) recommends as a common theme "interval history and physical pelvic examination every 3 months in the initial 2 years following definitive treatment. Physician visits are increased to once every 6 months in the subsequent 3 years. Once patient completes 5 years of regular follow-up then further plan is individualized according to individual risk (most commonly being once every year). There is no definite opinion on maximum duration of follow-up though many clinicians may choose to follow up life-long or at least till 10 years." Also, if a patient defaults on follow-up then, threshold for requesting additional investigations on next subsequent visit is lowered.

The following discussion summarizes the unique aspects of follow-up/surveillance protocols for common gynecologic malignancies following definitive primary treatment.

CERVICAL CANCER

Despite being a preventable malignancy and Government National Cancer Control Screening Program, majority of patients continue to present at an advanced stage in India. Fortunately, its incidence has shown a declining trend of late yet, it remains the second most common cancer afflicting Indian women and claims more than 65,000 lives every year.[2] Patients are followed up by the standard schedule mentioned previously. There is controversy on utility of vaginal/cervical cytology in the follow-up setting for detecting recurrent cervical cancer and guidelines allow clinicians to individualize this decision with stakeholders being made aware of the fact that likelihood of detecting an asymptomatic recurrence by this method alone is low. Imaging and laboratory investigations (usually limited to complete blood count and renal function test) should be individualized based on symptoms and findings of clinical examination. Fortunately, majority of recurrences in cervical cancers can be salvaged and are symptomatic at presentation. In our institute, we perform

X-ray chest, ultrasound abdomen and pelvis, and vault smear at every visit as a routine.

EPITHELIAL OVARIAN CANCER, FALLOPIAN TUBE CANCER, PRIMARY PERITONEAL CANCER

Recurrent disease may be evident clinically (symptoms such as pelvic pain, weight loss, bloating, early satiety, obstruction, fatigue), biochemically (CA-125) or radiologically. Apart from standard schedule of follow-up visits, evidence for advantage of CA-125 (or other tumor markers) testing is controversial because a multi-institutional European trial found decreased quality of life and no survival advantage to treatment of asymptomatic CA-125 recurrences.[3] Presently, Society of Gynecologic Oncology (SGO) recommends follow-up CA-125 (or other tumor marker) testing as optional with NCCN recommending it among those, in whom it was elevated previously. For less common ovarian histology such as germ cell tumors, tumor marker surveillance is not recommended beyond 2 years if they were previously normal. Sex-cord stromal tumors are at a higher risk for recurrence and biochemical tumor marker as well as physical examination surveillance is continued every 6 months even after 3 years of follow-up.[4] Markers other than CA-125 that need to be individualized include inhibin, beta-human chorionic gonadotropin, lactate dehydrogenase, alpha-fetoprotein and carcinoembryonic antigen. Genetic risk evaluation and counseling should be offered at some point in follow-up, if it was not done previously. The common genes targeted for genetic evaluation include BRCA1, BRCA2 and BRIP1. Multigene testing by next-generation sequencing platform should be offered, if conventional testing for suspected genes is negative and strong suspicion for familial carcinoma remains. BRCA-associated ovarian cancers are usually epithelial, non-mucinous histology while Lynch syndrome may have association with both mucinous and non-mucinous epithelial tumors. Certain specific non-epithelial ovarian cancers can be associated with rare syndromes, for e.g., sex-cord tumors with annular tubules can be associated with Peutz-Jeghers syndrome or Sertoli-Leydig tumors may be associated with DICER1-related disorders. Imaging and laboratory investigations (usually limited to complete blood count and renal function test) should be individualized based on symptoms and findings of clinical examination. In our institute, we perform X-ray chest, ultrasound abdomen and pelvis, CA-125, and vault smear at every visit as a routine. If additional imaging is needed then, we prefer whole body FDG PET-CT or MRI (with contrast) depending on suspected local pelvic or systemic recurrence. If fertility sparing option was chosen then, threshold for requesting additional imaging is lower.

ENDOMETRIAL (UTERINE) CANCER

The general protocol for follow-up of endometrial carcinomas is no different from ovarian carcinoma with the caveat that utility for CA-125 testing is restricted to those with high-grade or serous histology and should only be offered among those in whom, it was initially elevated. For radiological follow-up, NCCN guidelines recommend optional chest/abdominal/pelvic CT every 6 months for the first 3 years and then, every 6–12 months for the next 2 years for those, with treated FIGO stage III–IV disease in case, fertility was not spared. In case, fertility sparing treatment was chosen then, repeat pelvic MRI is preferred for patients with persistent endometrial carcinoma after 6 months of failed medical therapy. Usually trigger for requesting additional imaging includes abnormal physical examination findings such as vaginal tumor, palpable mass or adenopathy and new pelvic, abdominal, or pulmonary symptoms. Uterine sarcomas are followed up in a manner similar to other uterine neoplasms. In our institute, we perform X-ray chest, CA-125 (in whom indicated), ultrasound abdomen and pelvis, and vault smear at every visit as a routine. If additional imaging is needed then we prefer whole body FDG PET-CT or MRI (with contrast) depending on suspected local pelvic or systemic recurrence.

VULVAR CANCER

The general schedule of follow-up visits is no different from other gynecologic cancers as mentioned previously. Cervical/vaginal cytology screening for detection of lower genital tract neoplasia should be performed as indicated. There is paucity of data on follow-up for detecting local recurrence in groin after lymph node dissection however, there is data from penile cancers in males which proves overarching role of physical examination of groin with imaging reserved for those in whom, it cannot be reliably performed (such as post radiotherapy, obesity, previous inguinal surgery, etc.). Sexual health issues assume immediate importance after surgery for vulvar cancer and patient education and early rehabilitation including vaginal dilator use and lubricants or moisturizers go a long way in restoring normalcy.

In summary, there are only minor differences in recommended follow-up protocols by different authorities and readers are referred to a recent update on post-treatment surveillance and diagnosis of recurrence in women with gynecologic malignancies by SGO (2017) for additional reading.[3]

REFERENCES

1. Miner M, Esposito K, Guay A, et al. Cardiometabolic risk and female sexual health: the Princeton III summary. J Sex Med. 2012;9(3):641-51.
2. ICO Information Centre on HPV and Cancer (Summary Report 2014.08.22). Human Papillomavirus and Related Diseases in India; 2014.
3. Salani R, Khanna N, Frimer M, et al. An update on post-treatment surveillance and diagnosis of recurrence in women with gynecologic malignancies: Society of Gynecologic Oncology (SGO) recommendations. Gynecol Oncol. 2017;146(1):3-10.
4. Rustin GJ, van der Burg ME, Griffin CL, et al. Early versus delayed treatment of relapsed ovarian cancer (MRC OV05/EORTC 55955): a randomised trial. Lancet. 2010;376(9747):1155-63.